Partners in Healing

PARTNERS IN HEALING

*Simple Ways to Offer Support,
Comfort, and Care to a Loved One
Facing Illness*

William Collinge, PhD

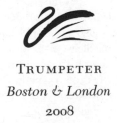

TRUMPETER

Boston & London

2008

Trumpeter Books
An imprint of Shambhala Publications, Inc.
Horticultural Hall
300 Massachusetts Avenue
Boston, Massachusetts 02115
www.shambhala.com

9 8 7 6 5 4 3 2 1

FIRST EDITION
Printed in Canada

♾ This edition is printed on acid-free paper that meets the American National Standards Institute z39.48 Standard.

♻ This book was printed on 100% postconsumer recycled paper. For more information please visit us at www.shambhala.com.

Distributed in the United States by Random House, Inc., and in Canada by Random House of Canada Ltd

Designed by Steve Dyer

LIBRARY OF CONGRESS CATALOGING-IN-PUBLICATION DATA
Collinge, William.
Partners in healing: simple ways to offer support, comfort, and care to a loved one facing illness / William Collinge.
p.   cm.
Includes bibliographical references and index.
ISBN 978-1-59030-415-0 (pbk.: alk. paper)
1. Alternative medicine. 2. Critically ill—Care.
3. Terminal care. 4. Caregivers. I. Title.
R733.C6515 2009
616'.029—dc22
2008017509

Contents

Acknowledgments

THIS BOOK IS AN OUTCOME OF THE SUPPORT, COLLABORA-tion and inspiration of many people over the past twenty years. I must first thank Laura Yorke and Carol Mann of the Carol Mann Agency for believing in this project; my editor, Eden Steinberg of Shambhala Publications, who provided helpful insights and wise counsel along the way; and assistant editor Ben Gleason, who so patiently helped pull all the pieces together.

Colleagues and life teachers whose inspiration contributed to the evolution of the ideas of this book include Karen Carroll, Abby Platt, Asa Povenmire, Janet Kahn, Tracy Walton, Janet Quinn, Laurel Northouse, Paul Yarnold, John Astin, Jerome Stone, Elisabeth Targ, Daniel Benor, Marilyn Schlitz, Jerry Solfvin, Ann Christin-Torres, Rick Leskowitz, Larry Dossey, Herbert Benson, Diane Wind Wardell, Susan Bauer-Wu, Ruth McCorkle, Len Duhl, and the late Venerable Ayya Khema.

I owe much gratitude and respect to the founders and staff of the Cancer Support and Education Center including Maggie Creighton, Jim Creighton, Karen Haas, Peggy Rogers, and Emmett Miller for their inspired vision to include partners as an integral part of the healing equation for people with cancer and HIV/AIDS. I am also grateful to the patients and families who attended the Center's programs, pro-vided many rich examples for this book, and taught me a great deal about healing.

I also thank the participants in the Elder Healer Project and the Caring and Cancer Project (formerly the COUPLES Project) for their willingness to be explorers in NIH research and help illuminate the path of self-empowerment for others.

Finally, I offer deep appreciation to the massage and touch-therapy practitioners in these projects who so eagerly and lovingly gave away their power by showing regular people how to access and use their own native healing abilities for others: Roberta Wentworth, Rachel Desley, Amanda Packard, Cynthia Garner, Martha Hamilton, Gloria Mallet, Kathleen Webb, Jeanne Colbath, June Kruger, Suzanne Reitz, Helene Royce-Toland, Janet Sullivan, Del Welch, and Leslie Wood.

Partners in Healing

Introduction

IT WAS A CLEAR SPRING MORNING IN 1989 WHEN I SAT DOWN
with a new group of eight couples at the Cancer Support and Education
Center in Menlo Park, California. They had gathered from all corners of
the San Francisco Bay area to begin a nine-week program that was on
the leading edge of cancer support, one of the first to actively embrace
an integrative approach to cancer—complete with mind-body medicine,
massage, nutrition education, couples therapy, transformational breath-
work, and bioenergetic therapies. But there was something even more
unique about this program: not only were the patients required to be
accompanied by a partner, but the partners were full and equal participants in every way, right down to the weekly massages.

As we worked our way around the circle with introductions, we came
to Jen and Phil. (To protect privacy, the names of any clients, patients,
or program participants to which the author refers have been changed
throughout this book.) Both thirty-one years old, they looked at first
somewhat out of place with their youthful attractiveness, as the other
participants were all middle-aged or older. But once Jen began speaking, appearances were quickly forgotten. As tears streamed down, she
explained that she'd recently had a double mastectomy and there was
now evidence of metastasis to her bones. With two children, aged three
and five, and a husband whom she dearly loved, she confessed a sense of
shame that she had been unable to summon up the hope and optimism
that she thought she should be feeling.

When it came Phil's turn to speak, he could find few words. Holding Jen's hand and his voice quaking with emotion, he simply said, "I
wish I could just reach into her body and pull the cancer out. I feel so
helpless."

Phil's statement made a lasting impression that I have been reminded
of many times since through work with hundreds of other couples facing
the challenges of illness together. Time and again I have heard partners

1

express a sense of helplessness and impotence at not feeling there was enough they could do to truly make a difference. Certainly they could provide emotional support and the many forms of practical help to make life easier—these are invaluable contributions and not to be minimized. But was there anything else Phil could do to actually reduce Jen's suffering, influence her illness, or even contribute to her healing?

This book offers a new vision of caring and its potential within an intimate relationship. It is written at a time of convergence of three powerful forces that together call us to reevaluate the meaning of "healing" and reconsider what we might be able to offer each other beyond the traditional limited conceptions of caregiving. These are the rising prevalence of chronic and degenerative illnesses, the parallel growth in the phenomenon of caregiving in relationships, and the growing recognition of the value of complementary therapies—not only in response to illness but also as potential tools of informal caregiving. The chapters to follow will show you how simple insights and skills drawn from the field of complementary therapies can be incorporated to make everyday caring for a loved one more effective for him or her while at the same time more satisfying and empowering for yourself. To set the stage, let us review these three forces to see what they can tell us about where we are and what the future holds.

Health and Humility

It's no secret that we are living in a time of increasing prevalence of chronic and degenerative illnesses. The most fundamental reason is the aging of the baby boom generation. A tsunami of seniors—or "age wave," as the gerontologist Ken Dychtwald calls it—will crest over the next decade as seventy-eight million boomers born between 1946 and 1964 enter their sixties. Millions of us are now well into the phase of our lives where signs of aging and growing vulnerability are the norm—not something to be fought against or denied but to be accepted and lived with as gracefully as possible. Added to this is increased life expectancy: the longer we live, the more time we have for the naturally occurring processes of aging and our hereditary vulnerabilities to find expression. Modern medicine routinely and methodically rescues us from crises that in centuries past would have meant certain death, giving us even more time to experience the frailties that naturally arise with an aging body. As the generation of cultural creatives that spawned the alternative health and human potential movements—with our noble ambitions to postpone aging and enjoy lifelong vitality—we now face the humbling realization that we may be as vulnerable to the afflictions of aging as our grandparents.

Of course, aging alone is not the sole contributor to the changing patterns of illness around us. Environmental exposure to a continually evolving sea of toxins and pathogens is generally beyond our control as individuals. Long-term diet and lifestyle factors add to our vulnerability, but likely to a lesser extent than heredity and environment. Whatever the causes—and there are many, both known and yet to be discovered—the net result is that today in America eleven million people are living with a history of cancer. Fully 40 percent of us are projected to develop it in our lifetime; this means that two out of three couples are likely to see their relationship touched by cancer at some point.[1] Other highly prevalent conditions include hypertension (sixty-five million),[2] chronic headaches (forty-five million),[3] arthritis (forty-three million),[4] heart disease (sixteen million),[5] diabetes (twenty-one million),[6] low back pain (thirty-four million),[7] Alzheimer's disease (five million),[8] fibromyalgia (six to twelve million),[9] and chronic fatigue syndrome (at least one million).[10]

An added dimension to this picture is that conditions historically associated with aging are appearing at younger and younger ages. As we saw with Jen, breast cancer is reaching more women in their thirties and even twenties, and other cancers are also increasing in younger age groups.[11] Diabetes and its complications normally seen in mature adults are showing up earlier,[12] and obesity is now epidemic among our youth.[13] Fibromyalgia and chronic fatigue syndrome, which portend lifelong vulnerabilities, are increasingly being seen in children.[14]

This is not to lament the modern way of life or the inadequacies of modern medicine. Rather, it is to frankly acknowledge the fact that the longer we live, the more likely we are to experience declining health. It follows that the longer any relationship lasts, the more its life span is likely to be colored by the experience of illness in one partner or the other—or both.

Popular culture has invested a great deal in promoting attitudes and beliefs that would seem to argue against this reality. We are told that we create our own reality with our thoughts and intentions, that aging is a state of mind, and that our own limiting beliefs or underdeveloped consciousness is the cause of aging and illness. The implication is that when the inevitable happens, there can be a sense of shame or failure, particularly in people who believe they have lived "right" and done all the right things.

By contrast, some wisdom traditions teach a more accepting point of view of these realities of life. For example, in some Buddhist traditions, there is a practice of contemplating certain "daily recollections." This involves remembering the following statements each day:

> *I am of the nature to decay. I have not got beyond decay.*
> *I am of the nature to be diseased. I have not got beyond disease.*
> *I am of the nature to die. I have not got beyond death.*
> *All that is mine, dear and delightful, will change and vanish.*[15]

These statements hold the paradox with which many in modern western culture now struggle. They speak to the inevitability of aging, illness, death, and loss. These daily recollections call for a truly realistic, *both/and* perspective. Clearly there is much we can and should do to promote well-being in our lives, and our actions do have consequences for our health. At the same time we should remember that ultimately illness is not an aberration or a mistake, but is an intrinsic aspect of being alive. To grasp this understanding may help make possible a more mature and accepting stance toward illness when it does arise—both in ourselves and in others. This awareness can foster compassion for ourselves and others rather than doubt, shame, or disappointment.

A New Age of Caring

There is plenty of evidence that a long-term intimate relationship has a protective effect on health. This shows up in lower rates of death from all causes. For example, in a study of a hundred thousand cancer deaths, people who had never been married—and divorced men but not divorced women—were represented at a 15 percent higher rate than people who were married at the time of death.[16] Another large study of ninety-four thousand people found singles to have a higher rate of death from all illnesses than married people.[17] And a study of nearly eight thousand men who were followed for eleven years found that those who got divorced during the period had increased risk of death from cardiovascular disease.[18]

Studies like these and many others seem to endorse the principle that living with a partner is an important influence on health and survival. This may be due to the buffering effects of interpersonal social support in helping one reduce the damaging impact of stress on health. It may be due to partnership's encouraging a healthier diet or lifestyle. Or it may be that people who are in an intimate partnership have other psychological benefits that translate into greater physical well-being or resistance to illness.

Whenever illness enters the picture, however, a new set of challenges and dynamics comes into play. Caregiving is now a central theme in many people's daily experience. The rising prevalence of chronic illness is paralleled by a rise in the numbers of partners and family members who provide some form of supportive care. A national survey in 2000 found that more than a quarter of adults were either in a caregiving role or had been within the past year, a number sure to be higher now.[19]

Spiraling health care costs and efforts to reduce the length of hospitalizations have created a situation in which many forms of care historically supplied by nurses now fall to partners—regardless of whether they are prepared. Those in a caregiving role increasingly find themselves attempting to deliver unfamiliar complex care and struggling to help manage the side effects of treatment.[20]

As a mushrooming phenomenon in the general population, caregiving is now taking many couples into unfamiliar territory. One of the most frequent sentiments I hear in couples' workshops and retreats was expressed by Betty, whose husband, John, had recently begun treatment for prostate cancer. In her words, "Not just one person gets cancer. Both people do. We're in this together." Caregiving partners vary in how soon they begin to feel this sense of identification and inseparability from the patient. Some are hit by it right away, while for others it may be a more gradual realization. In any case, it is more than just a subjective feeling.

Caregiving brings with it certain vulnerabilities but also some real potentials for benefit. There are risks of emotional and even physical depletion, but there are also opportunities for a heightened sense of satisfaction and fulfillment through the role of caring. In my experience, whether a partner becomes depleted or is able to thrive as a caregiver is determined in large part by two things: self-care and self-efficacy. Those who sacrifice their own needs in order to concentrate on giving do not do as well as those who find a way to care for their own needs and maintain a sense of harmony and balance in their own lives while still giving. And those who have a sense of self-efficacy, or *confidence in their ability to do things that make a difference* for their loved one, do better than those who feel they can only be a passive witness to their partner's suffering. Partners who manage to care for themselves and also learn ways of helping and building their sense of self-efficacy can actually thrive in a caring role.

We saw this in the Caring and Cancer Project, a study sponsored by the National Cancer Institute in which we taught partners simple massage and touch therapy skills for the comfort of cancer patients. In our focus groups before the instruction, many partners felt stifled by their concerns over when and how they could safely use touch as a form of support, for fear of causing pain, complications, or worse—spreading the cancer. With a little instruction and education, these concerns were eliminated and the partners' self-efficacy skyrocketed—as did patients' satisfaction with the renewed presence of touch in their relationship.[21] Hence the mission of this book: to empower partners with understanding and tools that will help them build efficacy and find satisfaction in providing support.

THE UPSIDE OF CARING

Mary and John live in a small, isolated split-log home in the backwoods of New Hampshire. They had met over forty years ago as schoolteachers and had retired to their long-sought forest sanctuary shortly before his medical problems began. Soon John had a severe stroke, and this was followed by complications of diabetes. Eventually he became blind, deaf, unable to speak, and had both legs amputated below the knee. They were now using home hospice services, with Mary as his full-time caretaker.

I had the opportunity to accompany their hospice social worker on a home visit to assess how they were doing with services. During the long drive deep into the woods to their home, I was struck by their isolation and wondered how they could possibly be managing so far away from family, friends, or services—particularly during the harsh and snowy winters.

We were greeted by a familiar scene. As is often the case in home hospice situations, the living room had become John's domain, with one side of his bed tight against the wall and the other protected by a high rail. Much of the rest of the room was organized with various rolling cabinets and boxes of care supplies interspersed with a comfortable sofa, a couple of recliners, and a fireplace. The picture window looked out onto woods and wetland.

One could imagine how easily a caregiver in a situation like this could feel trapped and overwhelmed and succumb to depression, addiction, or worse. And yet, after a year and a half, Mary exuded a most peaceful, relaxed, and radiant presence. "There is nowhere else I would rather be," she said, and it was clear to me that this was true.

The thought of moving John to a hospice where she could visit him daily and be relieved of the responsibility for his care was something she had considered in depth, but she decided that her life now was about being with him here and providing the care herself. My sense was that she was here not out of desperate clinging or denial but as a conscious choice based on what was personally the most fulfilling way she could live. She expressed openness to and gratitude for the social worker's arranging a weekly respite day for her and also an evening off when she could attend town council meetings, but otherwise, she was at peace with the twenty-four-hour responsibility of caring for John.

I am not suggesting that Mary is a role model that people should attempt to emulate. People differ in their natural resilience and ability to adapt to the challenges of interrupted sleep, hours of vigilant attention, intimate personal care, and days without respite. A person may have the caregiving skills and the spiritual maturity but still lack the vital energy to sustain such a lifestyle, let alone the economic freedom. What Mary does illustrate, however, is that in the midst of a highly demanding situation, one can still find great satisfaction and reward.

This was indeed the finding of a study of caregiving conducted by the Johns Hopkins Bloomberg School of Public Health. Researchers examined the experiences of 1,149 caregiver-recipient pairs in which the caregiver was a spouse, family member, or friend and the recipient was a disabled older adult. The caregivers were interviewed about the care they were providing and their attitudes and thoughts about it. The researchers later followed up to determine which recipients died within the year after the interview. They did this in order to classify the caregivers according to whether or not they were providing what could be deemed end-of-life care at the time of the interview—which is presumably more demanding and stressful than care for someone less ill.

Those providing end-of-life care had been helping an average of forty-three hours per week, and more than four out of five provided assistance daily. And, as might be expected, they were twice as likely as the others to report feeling emotional distress (30 percent compared to 15 percent). They were also twice as likely to have experienced interruption of their sleep to provide care (45 percent versus 21 percent). Fewer than 5 percent of the partners had used support services for themselves such as respite care or support groups, perhaps because of constraints on their time and energy to find such services or a simple lack of other people who could fill in for them.

Despite these burdens, however, the end-of-life care partners still reported the experience to be rewarding. In fact, they actually reported *more* satisfaction and a *greater* sense of reward than the caregivers whose recipients were still alive a year later and who were providing care that was presumably less demanding. Sixty-nine percent of the end-of-life care providers stated that the experience helped them appreciate life more, versus 60 percent of those providing less intense care; over 70 percent said it made them feel good about themselves, versus 62 percent; and 76 percent reported it helped them feel useful and needed, versus 65 percent. All in all, while those more intensively involved in caregiving had greater challenges and strains, they were actually more likely to report rewards and satisfaction from the experience.[22]

Most caregiving, of course, is not end-of-life care but is geared more toward coping with long-term chronic conditions. In fact, even the term *caregiving* itself may not be the most useful way to describe what goes on in couples who have been together long enough for a need for increased care in one partner to materialize. It may be better described as simply another *level* of caring in a relationship that is already based on caring and sharing life's journey together.

If you accept the proposition that a long-term intimate relationship is a vehicle for personal growth and evolution toward more and more wholeness for each individual, then the term *caregiver* quickly diminishes in importance. Partners in a relationship in which caregiving is taking place share a mutual journey of becoming more whole, each in his or her own way, and whatever happens in the context of that relationship is grist for the mill. To the extent that providing care for your partner is a natural expression of your connectedness with each other, it is inherently healing and self-affirming for you to give it and for your partner to receive it.

One thing we learned in the Caring and Cancer Project was that even though the care partner was the one who received instruction, patients increased their own use of touch in the relationship. Somehow the permission and encouragement provided in the instruction fostered a heightened recognition that caring is the basis of the relationship and is not confined to the role of caregiver. Several patients who were undergoing cancer treatment found fulfillment and satisfaction in providing care to their own partner. As one patient stated, "It confirmed that you are supposed to have your hands all over the person that you love and care for. We've found ourselves touching each other more, being more deeply present to each other, and more comforting to each other. It seems like we are in a partnership of giving comfort to each other."

From Caring to Healing

Modern medical practice has evolved in recent years to embrace complementary and alternative therapies in an integrative approach to healing. The new paradigm, called integrative medicine, combines the insights of diverse healing traditions to understand health and illness and to find ways to enhance the quality of life and promote healing. Integrative medicine has proved especially helpful in treating chronic illnesses for which conventional medicine, whose historical orientation lies in crisis and acute care, has limited effectiveness.

As millions of baby boomers have voted with their feet and pocketbooks for complementary and alternative therapies in the last twenty years, funding for research on the effects of many of these approaches has grown markedly. The National Institutes of Health and other federal

grant programs now routinely fund studies into complementary therapies for some of our most stubborn public health problems, including
cancer, heart disease, and others.

One benefit of this has been the recognition of just how simple some
complementary therapies are and how little effort is sometimes needed
to yield major benefits. For example, a large study at Memorial Sloan-
Kettering Cancer Center recently found that a single massage of as little
as twenty minutes could cut cancer patients' symptoms and treatment
side effects in half, and in some cases these benefits lasted *forty-eight
hours or more.*[23] Any drug that could do this—without side effects, no
less—would be a boon for a pharmaceutical company and would de-
mand top dollar. And yet the techniques used were basic and simple
methods that are traditional in the massage field. In fact, there is no
reason to doubt they could be easily learned and regularly applied by the
partners of cancer patients at home, extending these effects indefinitely.
This is the mission of the Caring and Cancer Project.

This possibility creates an interesting challenge to our traditional so-
cietal attitudes toward health care services. After all, our conditioning
has been to defer to experts with advanced professional training and
certifications for all healing interventions. Our cultural model of health
care is that it is a for-profit business enterprise owned by experts rather
than a simple universal human right.

This professional ethos has been extended to the field of complementary therapies. And yet, many such therapies have their roots in history
that preceded the existence of professional training or credentialing of
any kind. Many therapies—including massage, energy healing, nutri-
tional and herbal therapies, and even acupuncture—trace their origins
to folk tradition, religious teachings, or family lineage. It is ironic that
the idea of empowering laypeople today with some time-honored caring skills can meet resistance from a few professionals or organizations
that claim a certain body of knowledge as intellectual property or argue
that the public needs to be protected from unqualified people learning
and practicing such skills.

A movement is now afoot to bring education about safe and simple
complementary therapies into the world of caregiving. The repertoire
of lay caregivers is being expanded to incorporate simple methods that

can make a real difference in patients' comfort and quality of life. Such initiatives are being taken by practitioners across the fields of medicine, nursing, clinical social work, health education, health psychology, pastoral care, and other disciplines who work directly with caregivers. My own research involves teaching caregivers simple skills of massage (the Caring and Cancer Project) and energy-based touch therapy (the Elder Healer Project,[24] a study sponsored by the National Institute on Aging) that can have significant impact on comfort and well-being. As I will describe in later chapters, we have seen real benefits for caregivers themselves from this instruction and practice.

One of the champions of this movement is Professor Ruth McCorkle, PhD, who heads the Center for Excellence in Chronic Illness Care at the Yale School of Nursing. She and her colleagues have conducted studies in caregiver training and have concluded that teaching caregivers to become proficient in the physical and psychological aspects of patient care will benefit both patients and caregivers.[25] In one study, nurses and social workers taught a six-hour program for 187 caregivers that addressed symptom management, psychosocial support, and resource identification. In the follow-up period after the training, the caregivers' sense of being burdened by their caring tasks lessened or remained steady even when the intensity of their caregiving responsibilities increased. Even more important was the finding that with their newfound sense of confidence and competence, *their ratings of their own health had actually improved.*[26]

How caring could tangibly affect a caregiver's health was demonstrated in an interesting study at the University of Miami School of Medicine's Touch Research Institute.[27] In a study of ten elderly volunteers, researchers compared the effects of receiving versus giving massage on psychological well-being and physiological measures of stress. Three times a week for three weeks, the elders received a Swedish-style massage. They were then given instruction in how to provide massage to infants. For the next three weeks, three times per week, they massaged infants at a day-care facility. After giving massage to the infants, the elders actually had *greater* gains in self-esteem and reductions in anxiety, depression, heart rate, and the stress hormone cortisol than they did from receiving massage themselves.

❜ ❜ ❜

The experiences of people in these studies as well as in the Caring and Cancer Project, the Elder Healer Project, and other adventures like them point to an important new principle that millions of caregivers are discovering each day: caring for another can be healing for you. To regularly access heartfelt compassion and to exercise your own innate healing abilities for your partner can bring you unexpected rewards on many levels. This book is offered in the spirit of empowering you with insights and tools you can use to enjoy your own healing abilities. Along the way, it counsels you in the importance of taking care of yourself first, before embarking on some very simple yet rewarding strategies for building a network of support, using simple touch and energy-based healing skills, exploring distant healing techniques, communication, and other means by which you can express your caring. By joining with your partner in this journey, the two of you can truly become partners in healing.

PART ONE

Putting Yourself First

1

The Paradox of Caring

YOUR HEART, LIKE ALL OTHER MUSCLES AND TISSUES IN YOUR body, has to be supplied with a continuous flow of blood, oxygen, and nutrients to stay alive. To accomplish this, your heart pumps blood to itself first—before sending it to any other part of your body—regardless of what's going on anywhere else. It nourishes itself through your coronary arteries, which branch off from your aorta immediately after it leaves your left ventricle. With every beat, your coronary arteries redirect blood back into your heart, wrapping themselves all around its surface like the branches of a tree and penetrating deep into your heart's muscle tissue to reach every cell.

By design, your heart is literally its own first priority. It has been since its very first beat and it will continue to be until its last. The paradox of caring for another is that you have to care for yourself first.

The Shadow Side of Caring

The metaphor of the heart gets at the crux of the issues of caregiver burden and burnout. Depending on the extent to which you affirm and care for your own needs, caregiving can be a blessed experience or an ordeal. It can bring personal satisfaction and deepening intimacy, or depletion and erosion of intimacy.

Being the partner of someone with illness can bring challenges for which you might not be fully prepared—challenges to your knowledge about how to care, to your time and energy available for providing it, and to your emotional resiliency if your loved one's illness is long-term. Recent years have seen a great deal of attention paid to the health and adjustment of caregivers. The most extreme challenges are for people living with a partner with Alzheimer's disease, advanced cancers, or other conditions demanding intensive daily attention or vigilance over an extended time. But there are many more conditions that may appear to be less obviously demanding, such as fibromyalgia, chronic fatigue syndrome, rheumatoid arthritis, multiple sclerosis, or others, which nevertheless can impact you in major ways.

Without adequate self-care, preparation, or support, the burden of adjustment for care partners can be considerable. One of the surprising findings of research is that their own distress may actually equal or even exceed that of the patient.[1] How can this be explained? Consider that one of the greatest sources of stress any person can experience is a lack of control—a sense of helplessness—in a difficult situation. Ironically, a seriously ill person may at least derive a sense of control from having concrete and practical steps to take, such as taking daily medication, having surgery, or other forms of medical intervention. All of this helps to channel one's efforts to get better and alleviate a sense of helplessness. The partner, on the other hand, may lack a comparable sense of concrete and practical steps into which to channel his or her energy. Partners who feel that they can only passively witness their loved one's suffering, and that there's nothing they can do to help reduce it or contribute to their loved one's healing, are at the greatest risk of emotional distress.[2]

Studies have found that partner distress manifests as mood disturbance (depression, tension),[3] poorer health,[4] and even lower immune function.[5] A particularly revealing recent study at the University of Florida looked at the long-term health of the partners of cancer survivors who had received stem-cell transplants. The procedure is quite traumatic for patients, and the recovery period is extended. Dr. Michelle Bishop and her team evaluated 177 couples an average of six and a half years after the procedure and compared them to 133 normal couples ("controls").

As you might expect, partners and survivors alike had more depressive symptoms, sleep problems, and sexual problems than the normal couples. Beyond that, however, the partners also had more fatigue and cognitive problems than the controls, and their odds of depression were nearly three and a half times higher. Further, partners who were depressed were less likely than depressed survivors to receive mental health treatment. They also had less social support and lower ratings of marital satisfaction, less spiritual well-being, and more loneliness than either the survivors or the control couples. The researchers concluded that partners of stem-cell transplant patients experience similar emotional distress and *greater* long-term social costs than do the survivors themselves.[6]

The point I want to emphasize here is to urge you to recognize the genuine vulnerabilities of being a caregiver and to honestly take stock of your true needs for support and self-care. As we will see below, attending to your own adjustment and well-being is a real and necessary contribution to the quality of your relationship as well as your loved one's healing.

How Your Well-Being Matters

What are the consequences of your own well-being for your partner? This is a very important question to consider, and the answer just might give you further incentive to seriously attend to your own needs.

Studies have demonstrated that there is a feedback loop between the two of you: caregiver distress can contribute to distress in the patient, which, in turn, may have adverse effects on the patient's well-being, adding further to the caregiver's stress. This has shown up in the work of Professor Laurel Northouse, PhD, RN, at the University of Michigan School of Nursing. She has found partners' emotional adjustment to be a significant predictor of how well women with breast disease adjust to their own condition. In her research, women whose partners were coping better coped better themselves, while women whose partners were having a harder time showed signs of poorer adjustment to their disease. She also found that each person's level of distress seemed to predict the other's.[7]

Aside from the partner's impact on the patient's psychological adjustment, another theme in the research is that in life-threatening illnesses, partner adjustment may influence the patient's actual survival. For example, when University of Arizona researchers looked at what impact the care partner's sense of confidence and self-efficacy might have on his or her spouse's surviving congestive heart failure, they found that it trumped that of the patient. In other words, while confidence in both spouses contributed to survival, the partner's confidence actually had *stronger* impact. Patients lived longer if their partner had a stronger sense of self-efficacy.[8]

How could partner self-efficacy translate into better survival for the patient? In their analysis of these findings, the researchers surmised that partner self-efficacy was a signal of *marital quality*. In the introduction, I discussed the idea of intimate relationship in general having a "protective" effect that translates into better odds of patient survival. Indeed, such an effect is one of the great assets of a relationship, but now it appears to be modulated to some extent by the *quality* of the relationship. Since you and your partner are part of one system, if either of you runs into difficulties adjusting to the realities of the illness, those difficulties may affect the other as well as the overall quality of your relationship.

One of the ways that adjustment difficulties weaken marital quality is through conflict, and a large study has affirmed a connection between marital conflict and patient well-being. The Quebec Health Survey studied 7,547 couples living with one or more chronic health problems. Patients who reported they had conflict with their partner had a more negative perception of their own mental health and reported higher psychological distress.[9] This would seem to reinforce the idea of a loop between adjustment in either partner and patient distress, and as we know, greater patient distress contributes to poorer medical outcomes.

Thus, beyond the general protective effects of being in a relationship, there is a continuum of relationship quality along which you as a couple can find yourselves, and where you are on this may even influence survival in life-threatening conditions. This principle was affirmed in a second study by the same team at the University of Arizona who conducted the earlier study on congestive heart failure. When they followed 189 couples for eight years, marital quality proved to be a significant predictor of patient mortality—to a larger extent than even individual patient factors such as psychological distress, hostility, neuroticism, self-efficacy, optimism, and emotional support.[10]

My point in highlighting these studies is that as a care partner, your self-care clearly has consequences that extend beyond your own inner sense of well-being. Self-care is your path to resiliency, self-efficacy, and emotional well-being, all of which will affect your partner and the quality of the relationship between you.

Essentials of Self-Care

MAINTAIN YOUR SOCIAL SUPPORT

One of the most basic principles of self-care is to shore up your own social support. It is well known that supportive relationships serve as buffers against the effects of stress, so that the stresses you do have in your life diminish in their impact on you—physically as well as psychologically. To know that you have the support of others who care about you will impact your own emotional resiliency. To the extent that you are receiving the support you need, your sense of optimism and confidence will be reinforced and your level of distress reduced—even under very trying circumstances.

This principle was illustrated in a study of fifty couples living with Lou Gehrig's disease (amyotrophic lateral sclerosis—ALS), a progressive neurodegenerative disease that affects nerve cells in the brain and the spinal cord. Because of its chronic and degenerative nature, it is one of those conditions that pose a long-term stressor for care partners. In this study, the care partners rated how much support they were receiving from others as well as the quality of their marital relationship. They also completed questionnaires measuring mood, caregiver burden, and caregiver strain. As might be expected, over time their psychological distress increased significantly due to the patient's condition. However, the strongest predictor of the amount of distress they reported over time was not the patient's disease status itself but rather the care partners' level of support and satisfaction with their relationships in their natural social network, *outside* the marriage.[11]

In a related vein, another study involving fifty-five couples in which a partner was undergoing chronic hemodialysis for end-stage kidney disease found that the care partners receiving high levels of support from outside the marriage reported the least amount of marital strain.[12]

We'll return to the subject of social support in part 2 when we address ways of building a web of support for your partner. There may be overlap between your personal network and that of your partner, but my point here is to emphasize maintaining your own personal web regardless of the degree of overlap.

TAKE ADVANTAGE OF SUPPORT SERVICES

In the Johns Hopkins study of caregivers, fewer than 5 percent of the partners had used support services for themselves.[13] And yet, some forms of support available from professionals or organizations can make a huge difference for you. A therapist, counselor, or spiritual adviser can serve as a "confessor" and support you in many important ways that might not be available from people in your natural social network. For example, you may not feel as safe or comfortable discussing certain feelings, thoughts, or fears with a friend as you might with a professional who can hear all your feelings without judgment. It is entirely normal to have a shadow side to your feelings of caring and compassion, particularly if caregiving has become a long-term stressor for you.

To have a safe place to discuss how you are coping with the challenges of caregiving or to simply sort through troubling or conflicting emotions can be essential to maintaining your own sense of perspective and can help you keep in touch with your deeper values and purposes in caring for your loved one. There are also support groups and therapy groups that have this same agenda. Groups can be even more validating, as they afford the opportunity to see that you are not alone and others are grappling with the same issues you are. Many hospitals, cancer centers, and support organizations for specific illnesses have such support groups for spouses and caregivers.

Other services exist for more concrete needs. If you are engaged in a heavy schedule of caregiving, one of the most important but often neglected needs is for respite for yourself, either to take care of necessary trips outside the home or simply to have time to rejuvenate yourself. One of the great blessings of a well-organized support network is the availability of people to give you breaks of time, but there are also formal respite services in many communities. If you are in need of respite, you can find out about available resources by contacting the social work department of your local hospital, any hospice, or other community support agencies that serve people living at home with illness.

Depending on your eligibility or that of your loved one, there are often other forms of logistical support you may be unaware of that can be a real help. Examples are Meals on Wheels programs to reduce the burden of meal preparation, and transportation or prescription delivery programs. Despite the belt-tightening of human services in most communities, many innovative, helpful, and practical services are still available for homebound people who are ill and their caregivers, and I would encourage you to investigate.

I have seen that a common obstacle to caregivers' getting support is a simple lack of awareness of what is available. Another common obstacle is a lack of respite help so that they could pursue such services. Both of these issues require connecting with the right resources for information about what is available. The key people who will know about and can connect you to these resources are hospital social workers and staff of community agencies that serve people with illness living at home.

CULTIVATE YOUR INNER SUPPORT

You can find internal support through discovering meaning in or taking a spiritual perspective on your circumstances. Through working at this level, you can transform a stressful situation into one that holds seeds of satisfaction and fulfillment.

One of the first places people turn for meaning in difficult times is obviously their religious or spiritual faith. People who do well as caregivers tend to have a clear belief about what they are doing that gives their circumstances a positive purpose and helps them to derive a sense of satisfaction from caregiving. Such satisfaction might come from seeing your loved one through new eyes as a spiritual being or coming to regard your caregiving as fulfillment of a calling that deepens your own sense of alignment with Spirit.

The value of spirituality for helping caregivers maintain themselves through adversity has been shown in several studies. For example, one study of 252 cancer partners found that those with a stronger sense of spirituality had reduced signs of psychological distress compared to their counterparts with a weaker sense of spirituality, *even when the burden of care they had to provide increased.*[14] This was confirmed in another study with 403 cancer partners, which also found faith and meaning to have a protective effect on mental health in the face of chronic stress.[15] This study was accompanied by an interesting caveat about spiritual enthusiasm, however. Partners whose faith was particularly strong were also more inclined to neglect their own physical health when providing care. This could actually work against their long-term well-being and is a reminder of the importance of staying in balance on all levels.

Another way you can help yourself stay ahead of the shadow is through discovering personally meaningful benefits that make the sacrifices of caregiving a means to gain something you truly value—what psychologists call *benefit finding*. What can you gain from providing care? A greater sense of closeness? A sense of fulfillment? A sense of giving back? For many care partners, the most obvious benefit they notice is a solidification of the relationship, as if the urgency of illness propels them to a deeper sense of devotion that makes life richer—the "We're in this together" experience that Betty observed in the introduction.

Benefit finding was the subject of a study of 896 cancer partners that sought to explore what kinds of benefits people identified. Six recurrent themes were seen:

1. Learning acceptance of what has happened
2. Learning to have empathy for others
3. Appreciation of new relationships gained through the experience of caregiving
4. Heightened sense of family closeness
5. More favorable self-image as a result of service
6. Reprioritization of personal values

Not all of these benefits turned out to lead to improved adjustment in the caregivers, however. Those that seemed to help the most were learning acceptance and appreciation of new relationships. Two benefits that were actually associated with poorer adjustment—in the form of increased depression—were becoming more empathic toward others and reprioritizing one's values.[16]

What could be wrong with becoming more empathic? It may be that the increased sense of empathy for others led to greater sensitivity to their suffering at a time when the caregiver felt powerless to intervene. Those who found themselves reprioritizing their values may have felt ill-prepared to make the changes in life they saw they now needed to make. These are speculations, but the findings underline the importance of caregivers' having supportive friends or others with whom they can explore their full range of feelings.

TAKE TIME FOR YOURSELF

Perhaps the most challenging self-care issue caregivers face is taking time for themselves—for exercise, rest, respite, social support, rejuvenation, pleasure, or doing other things that are important to your sense of who you are. Many grapple with the perception—consciously and unconsciously—that taking time or using one's energy for oneself when a loved one is suffering is tantamount to selfishness or neglect. This judgment—or the *fear* of it—lurks in the shadows for many caregivers and seriously undermines their attention to their own needs. It is a difficult judgment to resist, especially if you are reasonably healthy and don't have outward signs of distress yourself. This judgment seems even more compelling the more extreme or acute your partner's condition becomes. Yet, to ignore your own needs can set up a subtle undercurrent of resentment that can eventually erode the quality of your relationship and undermine the caring that you do provide. It can also compromise your own health to the extent that you are less able to provide the care you would like.

This judgment is usually an inside job, and that is where the lion's share of the work needs to take place. But it can also come from outside—from relatives, friends, health care providers, or even your partner. No one outside yourself, however, can truly know your internal experience or truly appreciate your genuine needs. Just because others may not recognize or understand your needs does not mean they are not valid or do not warrant your time and energy.

Ideally, you will have the support of your partner and others who have experienced the shadow side of caregiving who can empathize and encourage your pursuit of self-care, but this is not always the case. You may be on your own, and you may have to withstand the disapproval of others at times in order to sustain yourself. This may call for a special kind of courage, one that is seldom spoken of but is captured in the words of the contemporary poet Oriah in her book *The Invitation:*

It doesn't interest me if the story you are telling me is
    true. . . .
I want to know if you can disappoint another to be true
    to yourself,
if you can bear the accusation of betrayal,
and not betray your own soul.[17]

The time and energy you have are finite. To care for yourself while caring for another calls for finding the right balance and living it honestly and without apology. Let your heart be both your model and your guide.

2

Care for Your Body

AS WE HAVE SEEN, IT IS EASY FOR CAREGIVERS TO NEGLECT their own needs. The greatest areas of neglect are rest, exercise, and nutrition. Each of these is essential if you are to maintain the balance and harmony within yourself that enable you to care effectively for your partner and to cope effectively with stress. This is because each of these underlies your vital energy—it takes energy to care, and energy is also the foundation of your resiliency and vulnerability to stress.

To the extent that you are involved in more intensive caregiving, it may be more difficult for you to find the time to fully attend to the care of your body. But by taking into account certain basic principles, you may still be able to do more than you realize.

Rest and Sleep

A great deal of benefit can come from strategic rests or naps during the day. It only takes twenty minutes for your body to hit the "reset" button by interrupting its momentum of activity and going into the relaxation response. A "power nap" or even lying down for twenty minutes to just pay full attention to your breathing can have a powerfully revitalizing effect. You don't need to fall asleep and it doesn't need to be for an extended period of time, but it's best if your eyes are closed.

Remember that sleep is the very foundation of health. It is during the deeper phases of the sleep cycle that healing of both body and psyche occur. If your sleep is cut short or is interrupted, this interrupts those healing processes and sets in motion a cascade of events that diminish your vital energy and resiliency the next day. Do whatever you can to assure the quality of your sleep. This may include sleeping in a separate room, but other more subtle contributions can include eating earlier in the evening rather than later (so that your digestive system can sleep with you), having a warm bath or shower before bed (hydrotherapy), and taking simple sleep supplements like melatonin or a standardized extract of valerian (see below). Also, by going to bed before you reach total exhaustion, you assure better-quality sleep.

If you find yourself "tired but wired" and have a hard time getting to sleep, you may benefit from practicing the relaxation response. This is a bodywide state of relaxation that can be attained in a variety of ways, such as yoga or meditation on following your breath. You could take a yoga class or attend a meditation group to get some practice experiencing the relaxation response, and then it's like riding a bicycle: once you've experienced it, you don't forget and can return to deep relaxation more easily at night when you need to wind down.

Even experienced meditators sometimes have difficulty getting to sleep, however. While basics like a warm bath, a little yoga, meditation, or relaxation or breathing exercises can help a lot, sometimes more help is needed. Before seeking sleep medication consider trying a little melatonin, an inexpensive but surprisingly effective sleep supplement widely available in health food stores. Recent research indicates the optimal dose is 0.3 milligrams, not the 3 milligrams that is common in many brands.[1] Another option would be the herb valerian that can be taken as a tea or in capsules. Look for a standardized extract of 100-milligram capsules and try one or two.[2]

Move Your Energy

Get some exercise each day. Beyond its obvious benefits for your heart and physical body, exercise is a form of "energy medicine" in that it moves energy through all your energetic pathways, releasing tensions of both body and mind. It is a natural antidote to stress, a natural cathartic for stuck emotions, and a builder of vital energy. It will enable you to see your circumstances through fresh eyes. You will sleep better, and your digestion will improve, too.

Eat Mindfully

Maintain good nutrition for yourself. If you are skipping meals, not eating on a regular schedule, or not eating a healthy diet, this will all be reflected in your vital energy and resiliency. A valuable insight from

Oriental medicine is that your digestion is strongest at midday and weakest in the evening. Therefore, if you eat your heaviest meal at midday and a lighter meal in the evening (rather than the other way around as we Westerners tend to do), your digestion is more complete and your body better nourished. A lighter evening meal will also contribute to better-quality sleep.

Understand the Stress-Energy Connection

Because stress is such a common concern in caregiving, a few special comments about it are in order. We are used to thinking of stress as entering through the mind—through our perceptions. Stress and coping theorists boil this down to our "cognitive appraisal" of our circumstances and our ability to respond to them effectively. The theory holds that if you are confident that you can master your challenges, you have much less of a stress response in your body than if you fear you will be overwhelmed by them and won't have the support you need.

This "mental" model of stress is helpful in understanding the role of the mind in the abstract, but it is not the whole story. More basic is the impact of your vital energy. Your perceptions of a situation are very much influenced by your ego strength at the time, which in turn is very much influenced by your energy level. You have less ego strength when your energy is low than when it is high, and your appraisal of your situation will vary accordingly. With greater ego strength, you think more clearly and appraise your situation more accurately, and perhaps more optimistically. You are more likely to see solutions clearly and be confident that you can hold your own against challenges.

Your ego strength is weakened when you are tired, hungry, or are physically unfit, and this will downgrade your appraisals of whether you can cope with a challenge successfully. The unfortunate mistake I see many caregivers make is in not appreciating the quiet power of these influences in their lives. They may feel overwhelmed by certain challenges of caregiving that they would see very differently with proper attention to the basics of self-care. Much depression is frankly misinterpreted as requiring psychological treatment or antidepressants when in reality it is due to the simple depletion of vital energy.

3

Stay Connected

ALL TOO OFTEN, BECOMING IMMERSED IN THE ROLE OF CARE-giving leads to an erosion of one's own personal web of connections. You can easily wake up one day and find that it's been months since you connected with people in your personal network, and a subtle distancing or even alienation has set in. Just as caring for your body requires time and attention, it's important to your well-being that you also invest in maintaining your connections with others in your life. It's important to your spiritual and mental health, and as we have seen, social support is a buffer against the stress of caregiving. We'll discuss this in more detail in part 2, when we discuss ways of building and engaging social support for your partner. Below are some strategies for maintaining your personal web of connections.

Take Stock

Take a few moments to take stock of your personal network. There are two dimensions of a personal network that influence how supportive it is for you. One is simply the number of people you can think of who care about you: the larger your network is, the more options you have for people to whom you can reach out for support or nourishment. The other dimension is its density, or the extent to which people in your network are connected with one another.

Size is good because it gives you more options, but density is also good because it affords a greater chance that people can organize and act in concert on someone's behalf. You can have a large network, but if the members are strangers to one another, the fragmentation limits a sense of family or community and diminishes the likelihood of "team efforts" for yourself or your partner. You can have a small but dense network, and it may function like an extended family or tribe with a more intimate feeling of being held.

Regardless of what kind of network you have, engage it. Here are some suggestions for staying connected.

Plan to Connect

Use a calendar to schedule activities with friends so that your relationships are maintained. This added bit of self-discipline may be necessary to keep your connections alive, as leaving it to chance and spontaneity becomes less reliable as you become more absorbed in balancing your work life, caregiving, and other demands.

You will also benefit from scheduling yourself for participation in activities or organizations that you care about, whether social activism, professional organizations, or recreational pursuits. The point again is to put things on a calendar rather than leaving them to chance; otherwise, this is another dimension of your outer life that could erode through lack of attention.

Spiritual Community

Consider making it a routine to attend a formal spiritual or religious gathering each week. The structure provided by organized ritual and tradition offers a reliable and comforting holding environment and point of connection with familiar faces, some of which may in time become part of your personal network.

In addition to more formal, organized forms of spiritual gatherings, there is also value in joining a weekly meditation or prayer group that you find you can resonate with. This can be very supportive even if not a word is spoken. To sit quietly with a familiar group and share focused attention together each week can be nourishing spiritually and energetically, even without social-level communication.

Seek a Support Group

Find a support group with other caregivers. These are offered at many hospitals and health centers. A support group can go a long way toward validating your reality and your needs and provide you with encouragement to take time for yourself when it may be hard to come by elsewhere.

There is one caution, however: not all support groups are truly support-ive. Every group creates its own group culture. Some are empowering and uplifting, while others seem to reinforce a sense of disempowerment and victimhood. Go the first time as an experiment to see how you feel while there and afterward, and let your intuition be your guide as to whether this particular group is right for you.

Because cancer is so common a variety of cancer support organiza-tions are available in many communities, and many of these have groups for caregivers. An excellent example is The Wellness Community, a non-profit organization with chapters in larger cities, many of which offer an array of groups for different types of cancers, for couples, for caregivers.[1] Also increasingly common are organizations that support caregivers of Alzheimer's disease patients. Hospital social workers and nurses tend to be most aware of any support groups in the community for caregivers of people with serious illness.

Create a Support Group

If you cannot find an appropriate group, an alternative is to create one on your own terms. This can have real advantages since you can choose location, time, how the purpose and goals are defined, and even who might be invited. It's best to cocreate this with friends or acquaintances who share your interest. This kind of grassroots creation of a group can be empowering and beneficial, even if it remains very small. Having con-tinuity of familiar faces and shared stories from one meeting to the next builds a sense of group identity that can go a long way toward reducing feelings of isolation as a caregiver.

If you do choose to create a group, keep it simple. A good model for convening an informal and leaderless group is to center it around the serving of tea or refreshments, or for the more ambitious, a potluck meal. The group process can be a simple round-robin check-in format in which each person takes a turn to update the others on their experiences in caregiving since the last meeting. Make sure that everyone has a turn to update their story, but only if they wish.

The real key that makes support groups supportive is the freedom to express one's feelings or concerns honestly in a climate of nonjudgmen-tal acceptance by others. There also should be an agreement to observe confidentiality regarding private things people may share in the group. The main challenge that sometimes comes up in support groups is the impulse some people have to try to rescue or give unsolicited advice when they hear another person's suffering. Advice from others may be helpful, but only if wanted and welcomed. Thus, it may be a good idea to remind everyone at the start of each meeting—especially if there are newcomers—of the basic guidelines for participation:

The freedom to express oneself without judgment, no unsolicited advice, and confidentiality. As long as people agree to observe these, you should be OK.

4

Follow a Daily Spiritual Practice

JUST AS MANY STUDIES SHOW DAILY SPIRITUAL PRACTICES TO be helpful in coping with the stresses and challenges of illness, so too can they help with the stresses and challenges of caregiving. Practices such as meditation and prayer can naturally lead to the relaxation response in the body (a natural stress reducer), and they can also help you maintain a clear mind and a mental perspective that makes your role as a caregiver tolerable and meaningful.

Any practice is worthwhile that helps you feel a sense of connection with your inner spiritual resources, however you may think of them. There are of course hundreds of ways you can do this, from taking a quiet walk each day to reading spiritual or religious literature, using breathing exercises, progressive relaxation, imagery, qigong, or traditional practices of meditation and prayer. I would like to emphasize that it does not matter so much what you choose as that you do something that you find satisfying. As with other forms of self-care, you may need to assertively claim the time and energy for yourself, but it will be well worth it—both for you and your partner.

Since meditation and prayer are especially familiar forms of spiritual practice for many people, below are a few examples of popular practices to consider.

Sitting Meditation

Meditation uses the mind to calm the mind. In effect, you are using your mental intention to direct the attention of your mind onto your breath, a word, a phrase, a sound, or some other object of focus, as a means to become more fully present in the moment and free from the stream of consciousness that normally preoccupies your mind. Most traditions of meditation encourage an attitude of nonreactivity and nonjudgmental awareness toward whatever is happening within you or around you, giving yourself a break from the agendas, judgments, worries, and distractions of your mind.

One of the most basic ways to approach this is through a simple breathing meditation. This is the basis of traditional mindfulness meditation (also known as *vipassana*), in which you follow the sensation of each in-breath and each out-breath for a period of time and return to that sensation each time you notice that your mind has wandered into thought. There are many variations in terms of what the object of focus might be and other aspects of technique, but they all seem to share the common goal of taking a respite from the mind—which, after all, can be a welcome relief.

For caregivers, there are two great benefits of meditation. One is the simple experience of relaxation of mind and body that it can bring. This helps not only to reduce the effects of stress but also to enhance clarity of mind and rejuvenate energy.

The other benefit is that it affords an opportunity to feel in touch with spirit. Whether you experience it as your own inner spirit or a spirit source beyond you, you can feel more connected to and supported by something beyond yourself through meditation.

Loving-Kindness Meditation

Loving-kindness meditation, also known as *Metta,* is a traditional Buddhist practice for invoking compassion and positive intentions toward oneself and other beings. It is usually taught in a form that begins with a focus on oneself, then extends the focus outward to others, then returns to oneself, then back to others, and so on for a number of times. Verbalizing the words serves to affirm and crystallize the intentions behind them. For example:

> May I be peaceful.
> May I be happy.
> May I be well.
> May I be safe.
> May I be free from suffering.
>
> May all beings be peaceful.
> May all beings be happy.

May all beings be well.
May all beings be safe.
May all beings be free from suffering.

This can be a very comforting practice in itself, and, of course, your partner is included in the reference to "all beings." However, you can also adapt the form to focus on your partner by replacing "all beings" with his or her name, as in:

May John be peaceful.
May he be happy.
May he be well.
May he be safe.
May he be free from suffering.

While doing so, you may also want to visualize your partner in front of you receiving these good wishes.

You could also expand the form still further and include all three levels—sending loving-kindness to yourself, then to your partner, then to all beings, and then returning to yourself and cycling through again.

This can be a helpful way to strengthen compassion for your partner and also to overcome any feelings of animosity that might develop from time to time. You might practice breathing fully through the repetition of each phrase, using each out-breath to send compassion and loving-kindness into the world. Try to experience the words deeply and practice making the intention behind them as full, rich, and sincere as you can.

Imagine joining with all of these other hearts, strengthening a field of loving-kindness that surrounds the earth.

A "Receiving" Meditation

At this moment all around the world, there are millions of people—from monks in caves, to nuns and priests, imams, students, prisoners, children, farmers, scientists, factory workers, and people from all walks of life—praying prayers of healing and goodwill for all beings and practicing loving-kindness meditation directed to all beings. This global field of collective intention is present all through your day, every day, whether you are aware of it or not. It's interesting to consider the fact that you and your partner are each included as recipients of all these people's intentions.

Take whatever posture or position you like to use for meditation, center yourself, and imagine receiving all these good wishes that are intended for you. You might use your breath as an aid to imagine breathing these good intentions into yourself through your heart. With each breath, imagine that this positive support is coming in and bringing light and love throughout your being, bringing light wherever there is darkness and healing wherever it is needed.

You might also observe to see whether you have any reluctance to accept these good wishes or whether you harbor any sense of unworthiness. If you do sense any such resistance, continue breathing in anyway and imagine it slowly dissolving in the light of the gifts you are receiving.

Daily Prayer

In daily prayers, there is virtue in familiarity. The more familiar the words, the less you have to think about what comes next and the easier it is to dive deeper into their meaning as you say them. There are many beautiful and powerful prayers to which you might feel drawn depending on your preferred tradition, from the Lord's Prayer to the Heart Sutra and beyond.

Some comfort also comes from knowing that such prayers have been uttered countless times before, and you are adding to a long tradition by repeating them now. Many people find the speaking of a traditional prayer a more satisfying practice than simple meditation, with the challenges of the wandering mind that it entails. Still others like to combine prayer and meditation in their practice. The distinction has been expressed this way: "Prayer is when you talk to God, and meditation is when God talks to you."

A particularly popular prayer that resonates for many caregivers is the Peace Prayer. This is often attributed to Saint Francis of Assisi, though its true origin is likely more modern, as it was first seen handwritten in 1915.

> Lord, make me an instrument of Thy peace;
> where there is hatred, let me sow love;

where there is injury, pardon;
where there is doubt, faith;
where there is despair, hope;
where there is darkness, light;
and where there is sadness, joy.
O Divine Master,
grant that I may not so much seek to be consoled
    as to console;
to be understood, as to understand;
to be loved, as to love;
for it is in giving that we receive,
it is in pardoning that we are pardoned,
and it is in dying that we are born to Eternal Life.
Amen.[1]

It could also be a rewarding exercise to write down your own prayer that incorporates your specific requests for the kinds of spiritual support you feel you most need, in your own words. Having a personal prayer that you can repeat as a daily practice can be a source of comfort and confidence.

Explore Other Practices

You may have another form of practice that is as satisfying as any of the above and fulfills the same purposes. Some people are drawn more to forms that engage the body or movement, such as walking, yoga, qigong, or even gardening—getting your hands into the soil and working with plants can be an equally effective path to grounding, centering, and contacting your deepest inner resources.

5

Take Respite

MANY OF THE PRIOR RECOMMENDATIONS IN PART 1 ARE really forms of respite in a sense, as they ask you to take time away from your routine to focus on yourself. But the concept of respite has a larger meaning for people who are heavily involved on a day-to-day basis in providing difficult or challenging care to a loved one. Because the strains of such a lifestyle can build up and take a toll on your well-being, respite has become recognized as a critical need in the caregiving movement.

If you need time off from caregiving, whether simply for rest, for personal care, to do shopping, or to attend to other business, respite help can be organized for hours or for days. It is not uncommon for caregivers to receive a whole weekend of respite. You have three potential avenues available for respite help.

Call Upon Your Network

The first source of respite help is family members or friends in your personal network. This is one of the valuable outcomes of shoring up your social support, as discussed earlier. It may feel awkward at first to ask, but the more you are in connection and communication with your personal network during your time of caregiving, the more opportunity there is for them to recognize a need and respond with offers of respite for you. You should remember that it is not just about your asking for help; they also gain something from providing it. For them, there is the experience of doing something meaningful, fulfilling an aspect of themselves by meeting a need of someone they care about, which is rewarding in its own way for them.

If you are part of a religious organization, this may be another resource to find people who could provide you with respite. It is not unusual for such organizations to put together a schedule of volunteers who want to provide this form of support to fellow members of their religious community.

A note of caution: If your partner has a medical condition that needs some level of nursing knowledge in order to provide care, or a mental disability such as dementia, make sure that anyone helping in this way has had suitable training. It may not be appropriate to have a family member or friend, even a highly motivated and available one, providing care if he or she lacks the necessary preparation.

Community Respite Services

Most communities have organized respite programs and services. The most common are fee-based and are offered through home health care agencies. If you are using home hospice services, the nurse or social worker with your program will be able to arrange respite care for you that will be paid for by insurance or Medicare. Other places to contact are your local Area Agency on Aging or other elder services organizations, some of which have volunteer programs that offer companionship or respite services at home.

Many nursing homes and hospices provide temporary housing and care for the patient—known as "inpatient respite care"—so that family caregivers can have respite at home. There is in fact a special Medicare billing code to authorize payment for inpatient respite care. This raises a question for some caregivers of whether the patient might not want to be moved temporarily. It is a good idea to discuss this option with your loved one rather than assume that he or she would oppose being moved. Very often seriously ill patients are aware of the stress their caregivers are under and would advocate for their caregivers in this way if given the opportunity.

PART TWO

Building a Network of Support

6

How Connection Heals

IN THE HAWAIIAN HEALING TRADITION KNOWN AS *ho'oponopono*, there exists a practice that could be regarded as the epitome of social support. If a person is in need of healing, the entire community is gathered together around the healer and the person with the illness to support the process. But before the healer will do the work, there is one requirement. Everyone present, including the patient, must first turn to anyone toward whom they have any resentments or ill will and forgive them, resolving and reconciling all conflicts that they may have brought with them.

Only then, with the entire community healed, will the healer do his or her work. This tradition is based on an understanding that our connectedness with one another is implicit and that we each have a role, no matter how remote it may seem, in both the causation and the resolution of another's suffering. And not only are we all connected with one another, but our web of connections reaches back in time to all our ancestors. The process is a collective effort to release any negative energy present, transform it into light, and thereby make possible any healing that is needed.

Other indigenous cultures have similar understandings and rituals that speak to an inherent sense of human connectedness. But in modern society, we tend to place a premium on privacy, individuality, and separateness—at least until serious illness strikes and forces us to recognize that we are not as independent as we had thought.

Caring and Connection

For many caregivers, the first impulse is to try to take on as much of the burden as possible to make things right for their loved one or make things happen as they should. In fact, this is the genesis of the term *caregiver burden* that in recent years has joined the parlance of the caregiver culture in a big way. Originally coined for studying the cumulative effects of long-term stress on spouses of Alzheimer's dementia sufferers, caregiver burden is now recognized as a major issue for partners of cancer patients as well as people with other chronic or degenerative illnesses.

Of course, the number one antidote to caregiver burden is to share the load and not try to do it all yourself. If you happen to be part of a large extended family living in close proximity to one another, or are part of a tightly knit religious community with a strong ethic of social support, you may have a leg up on keeping the burden of caregiving under control. But if, like most Americans, your connections are somewhat spread out or not very extensive, you may need to think deliberately about what you can do to build a network of support for both yourself and your partner.

The good news is that most people do have an impulse to help. People gain something from giving—whether it is a sense of meaning, purpose, importance, fulfillment, or belonging, helping others provides satisfaction. You may need help with concrete tasks such as shopping, child care, pet care, transportation, or other forms of logistical support. You may need help in the form of people's giving their time, to simply be physically present with your partner when you can't be there or to give you respite. Or you may need support in other forms—whatever will lighten your load. You have a better chance of staying in balance if you can navigate the challenges of building a network of support.

There are two kinds of challenges with which many caregivers struggle in this regard. The first is our inhibitions about asking for help. These may take the form of a conviction that one should take personal responsibility and not impose on others. There may also be a reluctance to reach out for fear of feeling rejected, embarrassed, or humiliated if the request is turned down. Others may need to overcome a sense of unworthiness or even shame at not having an intact family system or network that is readily available as well as a sense that a request for help is an admission of this inadequacy. Still others may resist asking for help because they are ambivalent about accepting it, given that it may mean surrendering some control over the care their partner is receiving. There could be a concern about the quality or appropriateness of the care someone else might give, but it could also be a simple clinging to control.

Such limiting beliefs can be overcome by first recognizing them and then making a conscious effort to replace them with attitudes that are more self-supporting. Remembering simple affirmations may help with this, such as "I don't have to do it all myself," "It's OK to ask for help," "There's no shame in needing help," "I am worthy of receiving help," "If someone is unable to help, they're not rejecting me personally," and "It's good to share the load."

The second type of challenge is more logistical: knowing clearly what you need and who and how to ask for it. Sometimes the stress of caregiving, particularly in a heavily demanding situation or if your partner is undergoing major medical procedures, makes it difficult to anticipate and see clearly what forms of support from your network would be most helpful. This is where the counsel of someone who can advocate for you can be valuable—whether it be a hospital nurse or social worker or even a family member or friend who can help sort things through and communicate with others in your network to organize support.

Ultimately, a personal network is a vital resource that can make a huge difference in quality of life for you and your partner, and there are many good reasons to invest in strengthening it and using it. In the chapters to follow, we will explore several strategies for doing just that. But, first, I'd like to give you a sense of how compelling the evidence is for making such an investment.

A Look at the Evidence

A huge volume of research has shown that being connected within a natural social network is a lifelong factor in health and risk for developing disease. In terms of its impact once disease is present, however, natural social support (as opposed to support from a formal group or organization) is generally regarded as tangential to medical treatment. And, yet, the reality is that social support after one becomes ill can be a major contributor to one's health and well-being. Studies across a wide range of conditions have demonstrated this. Here are a few recent examples that illustrate the trends in the research.

Social support may influence outcomes for people undergoing major or long-term medical procedures. For example, a study of 87 bone-marrow transplant patients found it to be a significant predictor of both physical and emotional well-being a year after the transplant.[1] Another study examined its impact on the survival of 528 patients on hemodialysis and peritoneal dialysis (that is, dialysis of the kidneys or of the abdominal cavity). Patients who felt a discrepancy between the support they needed and what they actually received had significantly greater mortality than those who felt they were getting what they needed.[2]

Long-term chronic illnesses also show the important role of social support. For example, in a study of 1,431 elders with diabetes who were followed for six years, the participants were divided into three groups based on the level of support they reported at the outset. Compared to those with a low level of support, the risk of death was 41 percent less among people with medium levels and 55 percent less among those with the highest levels.[3] In 320 HIV-positive patients, social support was found to predict both physical and mental well-being.[4]

Social support can play a role in helping people live with chronic pain. This was shown in a study of 336 patients with chronic neck pain who were followed for six months of chiropractic treatment. Those with high levels of support were more likely to experience clinically meaningful reductions in pain and disability.[5] This suggests that the support they were receiving had an additive effect, enabling them to benefit more from their medical treatment.

A lack of support may be a barrier to recovery from complex chronic illnesses like fibromyalgia (FM) and chronic fatigue syndrome (CFS). A study of 142 women with FM compared their functioning to that of women with osteoarthritis. Those with FM were found to be more sensitive to negative or stressful social interactions and—perhaps as a consequence—to have smaller support networks.[6] This makes some sense given the neurological basis of FM (as opposed to osteoarthritis, which is a localized joint condition). To the extent that the FM women were more stress-sensitive, they may have had to limit their social interactions and be more selective, but with this comes the cost of having fewer people available to turn to.

In CFS, a study compared social support levels in 270 patients to those of 150 disease-free breast cancer patients, 151 people with general fatigue complaints, and 108 healthy people. Support was found to be lower in CFS patients and the others with fatigue than in the cancer patients and healthy controls. The authors concluded that lack of social support may be a factor in prolonging functional impairment and the severity of fatigue in CFS.[7] Another study found that social support determines the extent to which CFS patients could benefit from meditation. Sixty patients were taught meditation and then followed for a year to determine the impact of regular practice on their symptom levels. Those who meditated three or more days per week *and had strong social support* were 3.6 times more likely to improve after a year than those who practiced less. However, those who had poor social support did not improve *no matter how often they practiced.*[8] It appears that in this sample, at least, a personal foundation of social support was a prerequisite to reaping the health benefits available from regular meditation.

There's also evidence that people with autoimmune diseases do better with more support. In lupus, a condition in which the immune system produces antibodies that cause inflammation and pain in various parts of the body, a study of 554 patients found that higher support predicts lower disease activity and lower support predicts higher disease activity.[9] And in rheumatoid arthritis, a study of 264 women found that their overall health status improved after meetings with their natural social networks were organized to shore up their personal support.[10]

Several studies show benefits of increased support in heart disease. For example, a study of 279 patients recovering from coronary bypass surgery evaluated the connections among family support, living alone, and subjective health. Those who had lower family support before surgery had greater depression, anxiety, and hopelessness than those who had more support. Patients living alone did the worst: they had more depression and hopelessness initially and at follow-up had more chest pain and depressive symptoms.[11] This appears to confirm that support offers protective and recovery-promoting effects for the heart, a conclusion that has been reinforced in studies of cardiac rehabilitation patients. For example, in 142 patients, social support proved to be a significant predictor of better posttreatment physical functioning and health outcomes.[12] Another study with 41 cardiac rehab patients found that the hearts of those who believed they had greater social support available to them during difficult times were significantly less reactive to stress and they had lower diastolic blood pressure.[13]

Many studies have looked at the role of social support in the well-being of cancer patients. Here are some examples from studies of people with the two leading types, breast and prostate cancer: In a study involving 179 women with stage II breast cancer, researchers found that the level

of support was a significant predictor of a woman's degree of psychological distress and that a high level of support is needed in order to reduce
the likelihood of severe psychological distress.[14] This was confirmed in
a larger study of 2,595 women with early-stage breast cancer, in which
the women were divided into high- or low-depression groups based on
their test scores. The women's depression levels were actually predicted
better by their level of social functioning than by their disease status.[15]
In prostate cancer, a study of 250 treated men found that higher social
support was associated with a higher degree of benefit finding, which
is an indication of personal growth and better quality of life.[16] Another
study of 89 men found that social support after prostate cancer treatment may improve mental functioning by helping them talk through
their prostate cancer experience.[17] There is also some evidence that social support may extend survival time in prostate cancer.[18] Studies with
other kinds of cancer as well consistently indicate that social support
enhances quality of life.

SUPPORT AND CAREGIVER BURDEN

As I noted earlier, the concept of caregiver burden was born in the culture of Alzheimer's disease (AD) spouse caregivers, and that population
supplies some of the best studies on caregivers' needs for support. In one
study with 720 AD partners, the size of their support network predicted
their level of depression.[19] Another study of 312 AD partners found that
their level of satisfaction with the network predicted their level of depression.[20] And a third study of 200 AD partners found that the number
of network members to whom they felt close, the number of visits from
network members, and emotional support all contributed to their satisfaction with the support they were receiving.[21] The partners of stroke
patients have echoed the preceding themes; for example, a study with
232 partners found poor family support to be a significant contributor to
caregiver burden.[22]

Can natural support from family and friends be replaced by an arti-
ficially formed support group? There's some evidence that such groups
can help. For example, a support group program for AD partners was
able to reduce caregiver burden enough that nursing home placement
of the patient could be significantly delayed.[23] Unfortunately, the inac-
cessibility of such groups for most caregivers limits their usefulness.

There's also evidence that the benefits may last only as long as the group does. This was shown in a study of a weekly group for thirty-nine partners of stroke patients. For as long as it lasted, the group did result in reduced stress levels, but these benefits dropped off when the group was discontinued, indicating that this form of support would need to be open-ended to maintain these benefits.[24] Hence, cultivating your natural support network appears far preferable to relying on formal programs.

Considerations in Shoring Up Your Network

In part 1, I introduced the concepts of network size and density: the larger your network, the more choices of people you have that you can turn to; and the more density it has, the more the people in your network know one another and can organize concerted action. Density works in favor of encouraging commitment to a cause and can make for a strong and supportive network even if it is small in size. In the chapters to follow, I will describe some approaches to strengthening your network in both these ways.

But, first, there is another aspect of social support to consider. In recent years, researchers have come to understand that not all support is good. Negative social support, or "negative social exchanges," from members of your network can have an adverse impact on a person's well-being and can cause lasting psychological distress.[25] Before embarking on any network-building activity, you should first sit down with your partner and do an inventory together. Talk about who you consider to be part of your network and make a list. Then go down the list and note who provides positive support and who is likely to provide negative support—through efforts to be involved in ways that are not helpful and may actually introduce more stress into your lives. Decide with whom you would like more interaction and with whom you would like less.

It can be awkward to simply put out to the world a blanket call for support and then have to fend off certain individuals whom you would rather not have involved. If your partner is seriously ill and you are juggling the demands of caregiving with maintaining a household, you don't need the added burden of having to accommodate people's misguided or ill-advised efforts. People may barrage you with unwelcome medical advice, unsolicited but passionate recommendations for alternative therapies, or deliveries of food that you or your partner are allergic to. Here is another time when you need to be nonapologetic about setting limits with others and putting your and your partner's needs in the foreground. You will have to articulate clearly to others what kinds of support would be welcome and not welcome, and you may have to tell certain people frankly that while you are grateful for their good wishes, you have the support you need for now.

The network-building activities that follow involve making choices of people you want to include in your network. Again, it should be emphasized that choices must be made and not avoided. Join with your partner and decide deliberately whom you want to have included so you can enjoy these experiences and receive the optimal support for your needs.

7

Call a Tribal Gathering

ILLNESS IN ITSELF IS A RISK FACTOR FOR SEPARATION AND loss of connectedness with others. People may tend to minimize the impact of an illness by thinking of it as mild or low-grade, not highly debilitating but more of an inconvenience. And, yet, the symptoms may be just enough to subtly alter one's patterns of connecting with others in such a way that, over time, bonds weaken and eventually fall away—unless conscious efforts are made to nurture them. An arthritic big toe doesn't sound like a life-altering condition, but if it is enough to dissuade one from continuing with a morning walking group, it could, over time, lead to a real erosion in the quality of one's relationships with several people.

Obviously, a more serious illness will have more far-reaching effects on one's ability to maintain intimate connections, particularly if it is a long-term chronic condition. As we've seen, certain chronic conditions, such as fibromyalgia and chronic fatigue syndrome, are characterized by weaker social ties. The chronic pain, fatigue, and stress sensitivity associated with these and other conditions limit people's ability to get out and interact with others and have the human contact that is necessary to nurture relationships.

What you as a caregiver can do—in consultation with your partner, of course—is to take the initiative to bring people together. Join with your partner in making a list of people he or she would like to include, and have a tribal gathering of some kind. This could involve coming together for a meal (a potluck might be especially easy), a party, or just an informal get-together for tea. It is not an occasion for problem solving. If you need a reason to justify the invitation, there are dozens of holidays every month from across the world's cultures and religions that could provide the occasion.

Orchestrating simple social gatherings such as this accomplishes three things. First, it creates an opportunity for people who care but who are reluctant to make contact because they're unsure whether, how, or when contact would be welcome. They may be assuming that your partner wants privacy or that he or she will initiate contact when the time is right.

Second, it affirms for the patient a sense of belonging and connection with those who show up and who obviously care.

And, third, it will reinforce a sense of tribal identity, as those who come will connect with one another while there.

This may appear to be simply a social occasion, but in reality it is a potentially powerful intervention. The health benefits of social support for your partner are derived in part from the simple realization that there are others who care and who acknowledge his or her importance. This affirmation of having a supportive and caring network is a contribution in itself.

Bring your people together as often as you can. The more connected they are with one another, the deeper will be the foundation of support available to them and to you.

8

Many Hands, Many Hearts

THIS DISCUSSION APPLIES TO COUPLES DEALING WITH SERIOUS illness in which caregiver burden is an especially significant issue.

For some people, one of the obstacles to giving support to a couple going through serious illness is not knowing what kind or form of support would be appreciated. It's not that people don't want to help but that they truly don't know what to do, so they wait for a signal and often end up doing nothing. Thus, more support may be available from your network than is being received.

This becomes a matter of organization and communication, and someone has to take the lead. The place to start is to sit down with your partner and outline your needs for support. What would reduce your burden as a caregiver? What needs to be done that the two of you are having a hard time accomplishing?

Remember, people who want to help but don't know how need concrete guidance. There are many practical forms of support that are easy for others to give and would lighten your load. Here are a few examples.

Meal delivery is a primal form of support to give and receive. For some people, cooking for another is a joyful act that brings great satisfaction. It may be that your network can produce one meal delivery a week or one a day. Some networks have schedules in which specific individuals commit to providing a meal each week on their assigned day. The regularity of this is a delightful affirmation of connectedness and caring.

Transportation to medical appointments is another practical form of support. Even though you might have a car and be able to drive, you and your partner could still benefit from a friend or relative's driving you and being there with you, relieving you of the burden of finding parking and getting your partner to the entrance; plus there would be added companionship to support you both.

Help with child care, either outside or inside your home, can provide

51

a much-needed respite from those responsibilities even if just for a brief time.

Pet sitting or boarding may be a welcome form of support when you are needing to spend extended time away from home while your partner is undergoing medical procedures.

Shopping, housekeeping, laundry, and even gardening are other practical and concrete forms of support that are time-limited and task-oriented, making them easy targets for people to commit to.

Once you have identified the tasks with which you would welcome help, you could share this information one-to-one with people in your network, or you could discuss them in a tribal gathering. One strategy some couples have used is to designate a family member or friend to take on the role of organizing support, ideally in the context of a tribal gathering. That person could then do the coordinating among the other network participants, sparing you that added burden.

9

Hold a Healing Circle

A HEALING CIRCLE IS SIMPLY A GROUP OF PEOPLE WHO COME together to join their collective intention in focusing on the well-being of an individual or the group as a whole. The essential element is this focused intention for the highest good to prevail and for healing to occur if it is in the highest good.

Anyone can convene a healing circle; it doesn't require any special training or background. You can organize this for the benefit of your partner, either with a small group of friends and family or at a larger tribal gathering. There are a many ways to conduct one. Below I will describe two simple approaches that your partner may enjoy experiencing, one with hands off and one with hands on.

Group Healing Intention

Begin the "preparation" stage with the group sitting quietly in a circle in meditation with eyes closed. If you have a favorite piece of relaxing and meditative music that you like for deep relaxation or massage, you may want to have this playing in the background. A good approach to meditation for a healing circle is to begin with simply following the breath to help become calm and centered. That is, use the breath as the focus of your attention for the purpose of calming the mind, returning to the breath whenever you notice your attention has wandered into thought. The group might sit together in simple meditation like this for ten to twenty minutes before shifting to the next stage.

After this initial period of preparation, you (or someone else) can signal with a bell or chime to begin the "healing intention" stage. In this stage, people remain with their eyes closed but begin focusing their attention on the recipient of their healing intentions. Everyone can, silently and inwardly in their own way, focus on your partner's highest good. Some people may like to use prayer, while others may like to use visualization such as imagining your partner filled with a golden healing light, filled with loving-kindness and peace, or some other representation of healing energy.

During this time in which the participants are focused on their healing intentions, your partner should simply sit quietly and be in a receptive state, focusing on the breath and at the same time feeling worthy and appreciative of the healing intentions that are being offered.

After a prescribed time—say, twenty minutes—you can signal the end of this stage with the bell or chime. At this point, the process ends and people can open their eyes. You may want to invite the participants to share their experience—what form their use of healing intention took and what they observed within themselves during the process. Your partner may find great inspiration and comfort in hearing these descriptions from the group.

Applied Collective Intentionality

Another method you might consider involves using a collective laying on of hands. In this method, the group begins with the same preparation stage as above. Then, before the healing intention stage begins, the recipient will be seated in the center of the circle and the others will gather around him or her so that each can place one hand on the recipient. If the group is too large for everyone to reach, then those on the outside can place a hand on the insiders so that there is a continuous pathway of connection to the recipient. (If someone in the group prefers not to use hands-on contact, they can still participate without doing so.)

Once this collective laying on of hands is in place, the healing intention stage begins. In this stage, rather than people quietly doing their own internal process, each person will outwardly voice his or her own unique expression of healing intention for the recipient. One person may offer a prayer, while another may describe a completely spontaneous and unique vision of healing, such as the recipient's being filled with golden healing light or some imagery of the pain or illness leaving the person's body. Each person may take a couple of minutes to verbalize these healing intentions while the others listen and follow along in their own minds, sharing in holding the vision that is being described together. When one person finishes, the next takes a turn, and so on until everyone who wants to has an opportunity to put his or her own healing intention for the recipient into words.

This approach is called applied collective intentionality (ACI). It takes advantage of our ability to join minds and hearts together and create a powerful field of collective intention in which the recipient is immersed and that is difficult to resist, no matter how undeserving one might feel.

I was first impressed with the power of ACI in a retreat with a group of couples living with cancer. Howard, seventy-two, was suffering from metastatic prostate cancer and was living in constant pain despite the medication prescribed for him. He described the pain as "like two five-pound weights hanging from my testicles." We decided to do an ACI experience, with each person focusing on their own personal imagery of the pain leaving Howard's body. It took about thirty minutes to make it all the way around the circle.

At the end of this exercise, Howard reported that he was completely pain-free for the first time in months. Three days later, he was still pain-free.

We'll never now how much of this result was due to the power of suggestion, or whether some kind of transformation happened in his body. The field of "energy medicine" is based on the notion that pain and disease are, at least in part, expressions of blockages in the proper flow or circulation of life energy through the body. It follows that techniques that may alter that flow or circulation of energy may contribute to reduced pain or healing. We know from studies of hands-on energy healing techniques like Therapeutic Touch, Healing Touch, and Reiki that some forms of hand contact can help reduce pain, perhaps by altering the flow of energy through the body. I suspect that what happened in Howard's case was that the collective intentionality of the group, coupled with their direct energetic and physical contact with him, transformed the energetic dynamics in his body that were involved in perpetuating the pain.

10

Organize a Prayer Network

As you'll see in part 5, on distant healing, prayer can be a potent form of support. Organized prayer can have a couple of important effects. One is that the simple awareness on the part of the recipient that he or she is the object of others' prayers is in itself a powerful affirmation of the person's value and generates feelings of confidence and strong support from his or her network. The other is that for those who are participating in the effort, it strengthens the bonds of network identity and sense of connectedness.

You can organize a prayer network on behalf of your partner in several ways.

1. Use group prayer when you hold a tribal gathering. You or someone else in the group could lead the group in a prayer for your partner. An alternative is to invite anyone in the group to offer a prayer and go around the circle giving each person an opportunity to contribute his or her own prayerful intentions.
2. Ask people in the network to include your partner in their prayers each day and ask them to communicate to your partner that they are doing so. This again will capitalize on the support value of your partner's knowing that he or she is the object of others' prayers.
3. Schedule a time for the network to join together in prayer remotely. This way people can participate no matter how far removed they are geographically and know that they are joining in an effort of collective prayer at the same moment. You might organize this by making an e-mail announcement or, if your family has a Web site, by posting a schedule there.
4. If your partner is hospitalized or bedridden, you could organize group prayer by conference call. Several very inexpensive pay-per-minute conference call services are available in which people simply dial in and enter a passcode to join the conference.[1] If your partner

has difficulty holding a phone, you could use a speakerphone in his or her room, and if it is a hospital room, you can even bring a speakerphone from home and temporarily plug it into the room's phone jack.

Another alternative for patients who are unable to hold a phone is to use a hands-free headset (under thirty dollars) that can be plugged into any conventional phone's headset jack. This way your partner can be lying down and still hear or participate in the conversation.

11

Attend (or Create) a Support Group with Other Couples

IN ORDER OF PREVALENCE, THE LARGEST NUMBER OF SUPPORT groups to be found are for patients, second are those for caregivers, and third are those for couples. In my observation, however, group support with other couples who are living with illness is an extremely positive and supportive experience and should be taken advantage of wherever possible. Many couples struggle with a sense of social isolation because they may not be able to get out and do things as a couple due to the illness. There is something very special about being in a room with other couples who are facing what you are facing together. It provides a powerful affirmation of both the value of relationship and the universality of the challenges couples face when one partner is ill.

We saw this in the Caring and Cancer Project, where couples in which one partner had cancer met four times over a four-month period to explore and learn about how to use massage and touch at home. While the purpose of the project was to teach skills that would enhance caregiving and improve the quality of the couples' relationship, in the end many expressed the view that the most inspiring and helpful aspect of the project was simply being with other couples and comparing stories.

We did not conduct the project as a support or counseling group, yet the times we met were indeed supportive on many levels. As a participant named Roger observed, "The best thing about the program was that we did it together with other couples. We learned together. . . . It's very valuable to be in a group of other people who have a similar condition and to know you're not alone, because it's a very isolating disease."

I've seen the same responses from couples with other conditions, including fibromyalgia, chronic fatigue syndrome, and heart disease. There is a deep compassion that seems to be aroused when you are with others like you.

The chief places you may find couples support groups are at hospitals, cancer centers, and community support organizations that serve people with illness. Since cancer is so prevalent, many communities have non-profit cancer support organizations that offer a menu of support groups; some are site-specific (for example, breast or prostate only), some are general, some are open to a mix of caregivers and patients, and occasionally you will find one for couples only. The Wellness Community is a national organization with chapters in many major cities that offer such programs,[1] and many smaller communities have programs patterned after this approach to support. The American Cancer Society, the American Heart Association, and smaller local organizations for specific illnesses often have couples support programs as well.

There are two kinds of leadership for support groups. Some are led by a professional (social worker, psychologist, nurse), and others are peer-led. In either case, the overarching purpose is to create a safe environment in which people are free to express their feelings and concerns and be respected and heard by others without judgment or advice giving. You may want to visit a group as an experiment and see how comfortable it feels for you.

If you do not have a couples support group available in your area and you have the ambition, consider creating one. You could ask a professional you know if he or she would be willing to help organize it, or you could do so on your own. It may be that within your spiritual community, there are other couples who would like to participate. Even if you find just one or two other couples to meet with regularly, this can make for a wonderfully supportive expansion of your personal network.

PART THREE

Simple Uses of Massage
and Touch

12

The First Medicine

YOUR HANDS ARE THE TOOLS OF HEALING YOU WERE BORN with. Anatomically, energetically, and symbolically they are extensions of your heart. They can communicate the full range of your thoughts, feelings, and intentions without a word being spoken. Before there was massage therapy or any other "system" of hands-on healing, there was the basic human impulse to give comfort through simple touch. And along with this impulse, there has always been a reciprocal human ability to sense whether a touch we are receiving feels right or is good for us.

All traditions of touch-based healing teach the principle that your attitude and the quality of your presence are more important than any theory or technique you use in touching another. The best training programs tell their students that attitude and presence are responsible for 95 percent of the benefit, and technique only adds about 5 percent. While techniques certainly can help—and I will provide some simple instructions for several in the following chapters—they are truly secondary to the healing and comforting effects of the compassionate intention and presence that you convey through touch.

In part 3, I will review the benefits of massage, but more important, I hope to allay any doubts you may have about your own ability to provide real, tangible benefit to your partner through massage. This is a form of interpersonal caring that has been professionalized to the point that many people feel it is beyond their capability. And, yet, anyone with a pair of hands can bring true comfort and peace to a loved one without formal instruction. Providing comfort this way to your partner is what I consider a *bull's-eye* intervention: your partner benefits from the comfort, you gain satisfaction from providing effective care, and your relationship benefits from a heightened sense of intimacy and closeness.

While there are many systems by which techniques of massage might be organized, there are certain common benefits that all forms of massage tend to deliver. First and most important is relaxation. This is not

to be trivialized, because relaxation is an extremely powerful therapeutic state that supports all the body's healing processes. The relaxation brought by massage reduces pain by reducing muscular tension
and by softening patterns of tension in the body that actually maintain
and reinforce pain. Second, massage improves circulation of blood and
lymph and the release of toxins from the tissues, all of which are helpful
for nearly all health conditions. And third, massage encourages the flow
of energy through the body that is necessary for healing on any level.
Massage is a holistic form of caring in that it improves the interrelation-
ships among body, mind, and spirit. It is also an interpersonal form of
healing, strengthening the bond and sense of connection between you
and your partner.

A Look at the Evidence

Massage is among the most researched and best documented forms of
complementary therapy. It has been represented well in the medical literature with reports of benefits for almost all major illnesses. Scientific
studies have been published showing benefits for people with alcohol
dependence, anxiety, asthma, atopic dermatitis, ADHD, Alzheimer's disease, autism, back pain, bone marrow transplantation, cancer, chronic
pain, cystic fibrosis, dementia, depression, diabetes, fibromyalgia, HIV/
AIDS, migraine, multiple sclerosis, myofascial pain, neck pain, Parkin-
son's disease, premenstrual syndrome, rheumatic pain, rheumatoid arthritis (pediatric), scar healing, shoulder pain, spinal cord injury, and
stress.

In addition, massage has been shown to help with such diverse concerns as aggressive behavior, burn and wound care, intensive care, tolerating diagnostic procedures, recovering from exercise, going through
pregnancy and labor, and preparing for or recovering from surgery. It
has shown benefits for infant development in neonatal care as well as
rehabilitation in the elderly.

A recent analysis of high-quality studies across a wide range of conditions found the largest effects to be reductions of anxiety and depression—symptoms that commonly occur under the stress of living with
almost any serious illness.[1] What's more, these general effects were

strongest in studies involving *a series of massages over time.* Here is where you as a partner can make a huge difference: While most people might agree that a good massage is a wonderful gift of healing, very few people can afford to have it very often. If you as a care partner are able to provide massage frequently at home, your loved one can enjoy the benefits regularly, and there is evidence that the benefits of massage accumulate over time.

Let me illustrate just how far a brief and simple massage can go. A recent study at Memorial Sloan-Kettering Cancer Center in New York looked at the effects of a single massage on 1,290 cancer patients.[2] Immediately before and a few minutes after the massage, patients rated the severity of their pain, fatigue, stress/anxiety, nausea, depression, and any other symptom they had. A variety of types of massage were offered, from basic Swedish to foot massage, light touch, or a combination of techniques. Sessions ranged from twenty to sixty minutes.

With a single massage, the patients' symptom scores were reduced by an average of 50 percent—even for those with the most severe initial symptom ratings. Then, two days later, a follow-up assessment was done to determine the duration of effects. Inpatients showed a gradual return back toward their premassage levels of symptoms, but those who were living at home showed no such trend; instead, their reduced ratings of distress *had persisted over the two days.* The researchers also found that when people had repeat massages, the benefits seemed to accumulate rather than drop off after each massage. All three types of massage—Swedish, light touch, and simple foot massage—led to improvements. The researchers concluded that major, clinically relevant, and immediate improvements resulted from the massage, even in patients with high levels of distress; and people living at home had greater improvements than those who were hospitalized.

What I find particularly heartening about this for caregivers is that the techniques used in this study (and most other massage research) were not difficult or advanced. They incorporated basic forms of rubbing, stroking, and kneading that anyone can easily learn. And they don't even need to be done for long to have an effect. Some studies have used massages lasting as little as three minutes and found significant impact on relaxation.[3]

The Caring and Cancer Project

The remarkably brief time it takes to achieve benefits with massage has been affirmed in my own research in the Caring and Cancer Project, an ongoing program to help people with cancer and their care partners improve caregiving and the quality of their relationship.[4] Funded by the National Cancer Institute, this project is inspired both by the desires of care partners to have some way of helping their loved ones heal and by the mounting evidence that simple uses of touch and massage can have powerful effects against the stresses of cancer and its treatments. While the project focuses on patients and caregivers dealing with cancer, the methods and insights are general enough that they apply to people living with other health challenges as well.

The first phase of the project has been completed and was attended by forty-nine people with a variety of types and stages of cancer and their caregivers. We had a mix of ethnicities, ages, straight and same-sex couples, newlyweds, married couples who had been together over fifty years, and parent–adult-child relationships. Participants first attended focus groups to share their thoughts and concerns about using touch in cancer. We quickly learned that although partners wanted to use touch, they were concerned about not knowing how for fear of harming the patient. They were concerned about causing pain, spreading the cancer, or possibly causing other complications. There was also concern about knowing when to touch and not wanting to give unwelcome touch. Patients were concerned about not wanting to be overly demanding, yet they appreciated and needed touch as a form of support. Couples generally felt strongly that they are "in it together" in dealing with cancer and that cancer affects both the patient and the partner.

They then attended a six-hour workshop together in which the care partners learned simple techniques and practiced on their patients under the guidance of professional trainers. Each couple had its own massage table, and each shared a trainer with one other couple. The trainers provided direct hands-on instruction in simple massage for head, neck, back, shoulders, feet, and hands for the patient, along with Therapeutic Touch and instruction in safety precautions relevant for the patient.

Our main interest was to see whether such a brief experience could have an effect and, if so, how long it might last. And, indeed, whereas partners had been using massage just over once a week before the workshop, they increased their use to nearly three times a week, and they more than tripled the average duration from a little over three minutes to over eleven minutes each time. Their confidence in their effectiveness (self-efficacy) nearly doubled, and patients' ratings of the helpfulness of massage more than doubled. All of these gains were maintained steadily over the three-month follow-up period. We also saw indications of improved emotional adjustment and relationship quality, and for caregivers, increased esteem and a reduced sense of burden from caregiving.

To me the most eye-opening finding from this project is how little time you need to spend giving massage to your patient in order for your efforts to bear fruit. We did a detailed analysis of just how long a massage from a partner actually had to last in order for the majority of patients to rate it as being "helpful." The magic number turned out to be only three and a quarter minutes.

In the focus groups that followed, the participants reported seeing real impact from the instruction on the quality of their relationship. Maureen, a breast cancer survivor, stated, "I think it brought us closer together. I've always been one to sort of keep my own counsel and not ask for help, but in this case, it just made it easier for me to do so, and I think it has strengthened our relationship." Louise, an ovarian cancer patient, found it to be a stimulus for communication: "I became aware that I need to be more vocal in letting Charlie know when I'm hurting, when I need his help. . . . I've become aware that just because I know how I feel doesn't mean that he knows how I feel, and that in itself has helped our relationship."

Mark, a prostate cancer patient, also noted improved communication: "I think the program has helped us to communicate much better. Rather than quietly going our separate ways, it's helped us to talk more and to have a lot more empathy." And even though the project was focused on teaching the care partners, many patients, simply by receiving, picked it up themselves as a way to give something back to their care partner. Hank, whose wife, Linda, has lymphoma, explained it this way: "It has confirmed to me that you're supposed to have your hands all over the person that you love and care for. . . . We find ourselves touching each other more, being more deeply present to each other, and more comforting to each other. It seems like we are in a partnership of giving comfort to each other now."

As you can see, simple use of massage can be a doorway to healing on many levels. We have since produced a DVD program, *Touch, Caring, and Cancer: Simple Instruction for Family and Friends*, to make the instruction available to anyone who would like to receive it.[5]

Cautions

Massage has very few risks, and they can almost always be avoided by either staying away from problematic areas of the body or using very light pressure. In cancer, while many people wonder about whether massage could spread cancer cells, there are no documented cases of this ever having occurred.[6] Massage around incisions and scars may be beneficial, but it requires special training and thus should be avoided by most partners. Massage to an area of the body where radiation therapy has been directed could further irritate irradiated skin and so should also be avoided. Chemotherapy can lead to vulnerability to infection at potential or existing skin-breakdown areas, and such areas should be avoided.[7] Areas of neuropathy (nerve pain) should either be avoided or only very light massage should be used; some people with neuropathy actually find their condition improved with massage, and this is being explored by some practitioners as a possible new therapy for neuropathy.

Of special concern is massage for people at risk of blood clots. For this reason, massage should be avoided if your partner has a history of blood clots. Also, lymphedema (buildup of lymph fluid in an arm or leg after removal of lymph nodes) may be worsened by pressure from massage. Lymphatic drainage techniques may be beneficial, but since these require special training,[8] partners should avoid massaging areas of lymphedema.

The key thing to remember in considering massage safety is that the main benefits of massage—that is, general relaxation and comfort—are available with only the most basic techniques applied to only limited areas of the body, and even with light pressure. You can give your partner these benefits by limiting your contact to the head, neck, shoulders, back, feet, and hands. These are the easiest and most accessible areas to work on and allow you to avoid any questionable areas where concerns might arise.

Another possible caution is how comfortable your partner is with the idea of massage. Occasionally, people who have never received a massage before are uncomfortable with the idea but may be too shy to admit it. One possible source of discomfort is if the person has experienced some form of trauma or abuse in the past and may not be ready to completely relax with this kind of contact. If that is the case, you can always begin very small in a way that the person can feel completely safe with; for example, you could start by massaging just one hand or foot and slowly, with experience, expand to the back maybe another time. This was an important insight gained from a massage program introduced at a community mental health center for people with histories of trauma. It was found that after a series of massages with this kind of graduated approach, they were able to receive supportive physical contact from another human being again, many for the first time in years.[9]

The Basics

EQUIPMENT

You don't need a massage table in order to do effective massage. Of course, it's a plus if you do have one (a lightweight folding table can be found for under $150), as you can adjust its height and walk all the way around. It's also a little easier on your body, as you won't have to lean or twist as much to reach. That said, you can still have great results on a bed, sofa, or chair, as long as you carefully position and adjust your body so you aren't straining to reach (any strain will come through your hands to your partner).

Remember that you don't have to reach the whole body in order to achieve the relaxing benefits of massage. Your partner may be totally satisfied with just a foot massage—sitting in a chair opposite you with his or her foot in your lap, or even with you sitting on a sofa and your partner lying down with her or his feet in your lap. A particularly convenient way to provide massage is with your partner seated at the kitchen table and leaning forward onto pillows or cushions resting on the table. You can stand or sit behind your partner and have easy access to the head, neck, shoulders, and back. Turn your partner's chair sideways so the back of the chair does not obstruct your access to the back.

Satisfying massage can be done through clothing. If you are working directly on skin, you will probably want to use a massage lotion or cream to reduce friction. Creams are preferable to oils, which are messier for clothing and bedding. It's also a good idea to have towels nearby to wipe off excess lotion or cream during the massage or when finished.

COMFORT

It is paramount that you assure your own comfort and that of your partner throughout the massage. Keep checking your own posture and position to make sure you are comfortable. Also remain aware of your partner's comfort and help make adjustments whenever they are needed. Make sure that your partner is not too warm or cold and that he or she is able to move or adjust positions as necessary. You should have a free flow of communication about this so your partner knows that his or her comfort is a priority at all times.

Have a selection of pillows, cushions, or blankets for bolstering and helping your partner rest in a comfortable position. For example, when lying flat on one's back, it's often more comfortable to put something behind the legs at the knee. If lying on one's side, it is more comfortable to have a pillow or cushion to wrap one's arms around and another as a spacer between the knees. Communicate with your partner to find the most comfortable position and support.

CENTERING

Once you have the scene set and your partner is ready, take a few moments to center yourself. As I said at the outset, your attitude and presence are the main prerequisites for your partner to experience a satisfying massage. To center yourself, you can simply close your eyes; take a few deep, relaxing breaths; let them out slowly; and set your intention to be fully present for your partner. You may also want to remember compassion for him or her, or use a few phrases of loving-kindness silently within yourself to help bring your attention to your heart. Keep in mind that techniques are secondary, and there is no need to judge your performance. Your intention is to just let your loving-kindness and compassion come through your hands for the highest good of your partner.

Then, when you're ready to make contact, do so slowly so that you convey your own centeredness and peace through your hands. Every stroke begins with simply making contact. To do this, get comfortable, open your heart, and gently let your hands come to rest on the receiver. Before you move your hands, let them soften and "melt," so that they take the form of the body you are touching. Breathe. Now you can use a stroke.

STROKES AND TECHNIQUES

There are four basic types of techniques that are pretty intuitive and easy to practice. These are gliding strokes, kneading strokes, simple holding of areas of the body, and acupressure focused on a specific point of the body. The exercises in the following chapters show how to apply these techniques to various parts of the body. Here I will describe the essence of each one.

Gliding strokes (called effleurage by massage therapists) are long and slow, usually flowing in the general direction toward the heart and tracing the contours of your partner's body. Though gliding can be done with any level of pressure from very light to firm and deep, always begin with a lighter gliding stroke and only go deeper if your partner wants it and you think it is appropriate. A very light stroke would be like what you use to apply lotion. It doesn't even move your partner's skin. A light stroke would move the skin but wouldn't go deeper than that. Use enough cream, lotion, or oil with gliding strokes so that the glide is easy and no friction is created. At the same time, since you want control of your movement and don't want to slide all over your partner, don't use too much cream or oil. Your hands are always soft in gliding strokes, conforming to your partner's body. Long gliding strokes can be used on the back, arms, and legs. Shorter gliding strokes can be used on the face (the forehead, for example), chest, and feet. You can glide using the palm of your hand, your finger pads, or the length of your fingers.

Kneading strokes (also called petrissage) are the lifting, rolling, or kneading of the tissue. Kneading has been likened to working with dough. Any squeezing is done very gently—not pinching or hard, it uses just enough firmness so that you have hold of your partner's tissue and can move it as you want to. Don't use too much cream when kneading because you don't want to slip and slide. Rather, you want a good controlled stroke. Kneading strokes can be used on the limbs, back, neck, hands, feet, and chest. Specific kinds of kneading for different areas will be described later. In addition to these, you can create your own.

Always check in with your partner to make sure what you are doing feels good.

Holding is a very subtle but powerful way to give comfort and help ease pain. Another name for holding might be presence, because that is really what it is. In holding, your hands are still but they are not empty. You are holding someone you care about with a feeling of loving presence. Holding can be from underneath, as in holding your partner's head by letting the head just rest in your soft hands. It can be from above, as when you place one or both hands on an area and simply stay there, while you "listen" with your hands to your partner's body. You can also make a "hand sandwich," in which you hold a specific area above and below at the same time. The shoulder and chest (with one hand under the back) are good places for this. You don't need lotion or cream for holding, and it can be done by touching the skin directly or through clothing or bedding. Although holding may sound too simple to be effective, it can be very powerful.

Acupressure and other uses of compression focus on a small area by use of a thumb or fingertip as an effective yet simple way to relieve certain symptoms. Acupressure uses the map of the body's acupuncture points as a guide for where you can apply pressure for specific symptoms. There are easily learned points for reducing nausea, pain, headaches, or other symptoms.[10] This is a technique in which you don't move your contact in any direction except down into the layers of tissue in one spot. For acupressure, you locate the point you want, place a thumb or finger there, and beginning with a light touch, ever so slowly and steadily, simply press into the tissue and then release.

You can also use simple compression to press into a larger area with the heel or palm of your hand and then release.

The instructions in the following chapters will give you some simple ways to apply these basics. The world of massage therapy offers many other more detailed techniques, of course, but the basics are enough to provide comfort and satisfaction to your partner without the need for any special training. Remember that your attitude and presence are key and that the simplest use of technique can bring truly welcome and satisfying results with very little effort.

13

Foot Massage

FOOT MASSAGE WITH MASSAGE OIL OR CREAM CAN BE AN extremely pleasant method of stress reduction and relaxation. As with all the techniques to follow, you should always begin with the basics of centering and making sure both you and your partner are comfortable. You can use any of these techniques your partner likes, in no particular order.

Foot Spread

The goal here is to relax the foot by spreading it—from the center out to the sides. Have your partner lie on his or her back while you stand facing the feet. Take one foot in both hands so that your thumbs are on the top of the foot and the fingers from your two hands are meeting in the center of your partner's sole. Then slowly spread the foot by drawing your fingers out to the sides from the center. You will want a little cream for this, but not too much. Do this a few times.

Knuckle Sweep

Hold one foot by letting the heel of it rest in the palm of one hand. Make a soft fist with your other hand and gently sweep that fist down the sole of the foot you are holding from just below the toes all the way to the heel. Usually people enjoy some good pressure here, so you can go deeper than a tickle. You will want a little cream on either the foot or your knuckles, but not too much. Do this a few times.

Circles with Knuckles or Fingertips

With a knuckle, or with your thumb braced against your first finger, select a point on the sole of your partner's foot and press in gently, then make a few circles. Then lift your thumb, put it in a new place, and repeat. Check in with your partner to find a good level of pressure to use. Also place your other hand against the top of the arch so that as you press in on the sole, the foot is supported by the counterpressure above.

Milking and Squeezing the Toes

Grasp a toe as though you were taking a cow's teat to milk it. That is, hold it as though it were a rein in your hand. With your thumb and first finger, gently squeeze the toe, beginning where it joins the foot and working your way out to the tip. Do each toe.

Foot Reflexology

Foot reflexology is similar to acupressure in that it relies on applying pressure to specific points. It is based on the theory that certain points on the feet are connected to distant body systems and organs. It is an open question as to how specific the effects of reflexology might be on distant parts of the body, but this does not detract from the relaxation and pleasure that can come from this popular form of massage. In fact, several studies conducted using foot reflexology with cancer patients have found that as few as one to three treatments of ten to thirty minutes each can significantly reduce pain, nausea, and anxiety and increase relaxation and quality of life.[1] A variety of printable maps are available on the Internet depicting the geography of the reflexology points on the feet (just Google "foot reflexology").

14

Hand Massage

Hand massage is another very pleasant method of stress reduction and relaxation. You will notice there is great similarity to the techniques used on the feet.

Stretch and Bend

Stretching and bending the hand is similar to spreading the foot. Take one of your partner's hands (palm down) in your two hands so his or her fingers are pointed toward the heels of your hands. Now reach your fingers (of both your hands) underneath to the center line of the palm and hold the hand gently but securely with your thumbs right next to each other on the top of the back of the hand to help grasp it. Now keep holding the hand as you rotate your hands outward from each other so that your thumbs move a few inches apart and point away from each other. It is as though you are stretching your partner's hand open. The palm will arch and bend over your fingers, which are pressing up underneath.

Sweeps and Circles on Palms and Wrists

Sweeps and circles on the palms and wrists are especially pleasant with the use of oil or cream. Hold your partner's hand so it is palm up in your two hands. With your fingers under the back of the hand supporting it, and your thumbs on the palm, press your thumbs in and rub in circles—little ones or big, sweeping ones. This stretches the palm and feels wonderful. You can also place one of your hands under your partner's hand to hold it in place while you use the knuckles of your other hand to press into the palm and make big circles.

Finger Squeeze

The finger squeeze is just like the motion of milking and squeezing the toes.

Hand Reflexology

Similar to foot reflexology, there are also maps of points on the hands that are theoretically connected to distant systems or parts of the body. Again, it remains an open question how specific the effects might be, but hand reflexology can be another very pleasant and relaxing use of touch. You can easily find printable maps on the Internet depicting the geography of the reflexology points on the hands (just Google "hand reflexology").

15

Head and Face Massage

THE HEAD AND FACE ARE PRIME TARGETS FOR MASSAGE USING Swedish strokes and other simple techniques. The smooth tissue enveloping the entire head is rich with nerve endings and places where tension can be held. General bodywide relaxation can be achieved by simple techniques of attention to the head.

Head Holding

Head holding is a wonderful technique for helping someone relax and for letting your hands and your partner get to know each other better. Have your partner lie down with his or her head pointed toward you. You can be seated in a chair or kneeling on the floor, but make sure you are comfortable. Your partner's head can be resting in your lap or on a bed or cushion in front of you. Now let your fingers meet under your partner's neck and gently bring your hands toward yourself until your partner's head is resting in your hands. Relax, let your hands soften, and let your heart extend down your arms and through your hands as you lovingly hold your partner's head.

Head Kneading

Head kneading is a scalp massage that you give by letting your fingers press into the scalp just enough so that when you move your fingers, the scalp moves with them. Hold the head in one hand while the other hand kneads all over the top, sides, and back of the head. Then switch hands and repeat. You and your partner can decide together what level of pressure feels best.

Fingertip Massage

The surface of the scalp is rich with acupressure points that respond nicely to fingertip pressure. You don't need to follow a detailed map of the anatomy of these features. You can give a most satisfying form of relaxation and tension release by sequentially applying light to moderate finger pressure all over and around the head. By using both hands and both sets of fingertips symmetrically, you can apply pressure to ten points at a time.

Try to cover the entire surface area of the scalp with a series of brief placements of all your fingers. Your partner may tell you of specific areas that are especially pleasing to return to and spend more time. The temples as well as the insertion points of the neck muscles just beneath the back of the skull are often places where tension accumulates, which can be released with light to moderate pressure. Let your partner guide you as to how much pressure is right.

Face Sweep

The face sweep is a gliding stroke that can be done with no cream or a little cream. Sitting at your partner's head, place your hands lightly at his or her chin. Place your two index fingers in the space just above the chin and just below the lower lip, with the other fingers of each hand under the chin but not resting on the neck. Now draw your fingers up the sides of the person's face, coming all the way up to the temples and over the forehead. Repeat this. You can do this stroke with almost no pressure just gliding over the skin, or with enough pressure to drag the skin a little bit with the movement of your hands.

Brow Sweep

You can also sweep across the forehead. Lay your right hand so that your palm is on your partner's forehead and your fingers are touching the left temple. Draw your hand gently across to the right so that your fingers sweep across the entire brow. Now do the mirror action with your left hand. You can do this a few times.

Ear Circles

With the pads of one or two fingers, using light pressure, make little circles on the skull just behind the ears.

Ear Tugs

With thumb and forefinger, gently grasp each earlobe and softly "tug" while letting your thumb and finger slide off the ear. Do this a few times.

16

Back and Shoulders Massage

Gliding from Top to Bottom

As with any gliding stroke, use a little cream for this stroke. Standing at the head, with your partner lying facedown, place your hands at your partner's shoulder level, on either side of the backbone, with your fingers pointing toward your partner's feet. Let your hands glide all the way down the back to the waist. Then draw your hands back up along the person's sides. Do this as much as you both want.

Gliding from Bottom to Top

This is the reverse of the stroke above. Stand on one side of the table (or bed) at your partner's waist. Beginning at the waist, let your hands glide up to the person's shoulders, then out along the shoulders and down along the sides, back to the waist.

Circles

The circle is a wonderful motion on the body. You can do small circles with the pads of two or three fingers, or you can do large circles using the flat of your hand or your palm. As with other kneading strokes, use enough pressure so that the skin and other deeper layers move under your fingers. (In other words, don't just glide over the skin.) You can do these along the waist, the shoulders, or on the muscles that go lengthwise along the back. Do not do circles on the backbone.

Compression

Sometimes simple compression is the best treatment for relaxing a back. Standing by your partner's side, place one hand over the other on the back, lean in a bit, then release your hands gently and place them on the next spot. Don't stay in any one spot too long. Try doing it to a count of three and adjust your timing to please your recipient.

Kneading

As though you had dough or clay in your hands, grasp the tissue (skin and muscles below) just firmly enough to be able to lift it and release it—maybe with just a little movement in one direction or another. Get a good rhythm going with your kneading. You can do this at the waist or up and down one side of the back, or you can stand at the waist and knead the shoulder area from the neck out toward first one shoulder, then the other.

Cat's Paws

With your partner lying faceup, sit or kneel at his or her head and rest a hand softly on each shoulder. Press straight in with the palm of your right hand (toward your partner's foot) while leaning slightly to the right. Now relax the pressure of your right hand and press with your left hand into the left shoulder, leaning slightly toward the left.

Alternate like this, just like a cat alternately working its paws, while you gently rock from side to side. Use your weight, not your muscles, to create the pressure.

17

Acupressure for Symptom Relief

ACUPRESSURE OFFERS SEVERAL CONFIGURATIONS OF POINTS that you can stimulate in your partner for specific symptoms. Instructions for finding acupressure points are usually given in "finger widths" from a reference point—such as two-and-a-half finger widths above the wrist crease (away from the hand), at the midline of the inside of the forearm, to reach an antinausea point (discussed later). This term refers to the width of the *recipient's* finger, not your own. Your partner will also be able to help you find a point by telling you when there is a feeling of some tenderness or softness when you have contacted it.

The basic technique is to contact the point lightly at first and then gradually apply pressure until you reach a gentle yet firm contact. Apply the pressure straight down at a ninety-degree angle. Hold steadily for a few seconds and then gradually release pressure. Let your partner tell you what he or she is noticing. Do not rub or grind the spot. When you are ready to let go of the point, release the point slowly, gradually reducing your pressure until your thumb or finger is off the body. Never pull away suddenly.

General Pain

In the middle of the little web of flesh that connects the thumb and index finger on either hand is a point that when stimulated can help reduce pain anywhere in the body. Stimulating this point is known as "Joining the Valley." The point is located at the top of the little mound of muscle that puffs up when the person lines up the thumb and index finger side by side. You can press into it from above, or you can squeeze from above and below at the same time. There is a caution with this point, however: it may stimulate uterine contractions and should therefore be avoided in pregnancy.

Nausea

The point for nausea is called "Inner Gate" and is located two-and-a-half finger widths up the forearm from the wrist crease, at the midline of the inside of the forearm. If your partner flexes his or her wrist, you will see (or at least be able to feel) two long tendons in the middle of the arm. Press into the space between them (two and a half finger widths up from the wrist crease) and you will be on the point.

Anxiety

The point for anxiety is called "Spirit Gate." It is on the outside (pinky finger side) of the wrist and can be most easily found when your partner angles his or her hand sideways in the direction of the pinky. Flexing the hand this way creates a little recession just after the end of the wrist bone and between the heel bone of the palm and the top bone of the back of the hand. Press into this recession area and you are on the point.

Fatigue

The point for reducing fatigue is called the "Three Mile Point." You will find this point four finger widths below the lower edge of the kneecap and then one finger width away from the shinbone going toward the outside of the leg. This point may also help relieve nausea.

Headache

The main points for relieving headache are called the "Gates of Consciousness." These are located at the base of the back of the skull, immediately below the two prominent ridges, where the neck muscles attach into the skull on either side of the neck vertebrae. You will feel two depressions at these insertion points, and this is where you apply the fingertip pressure. You might also rub these points and the surrounding area for a few minutes.

You may also find it helps your partner to use the Joining the Valley points on the hands (in the webbing between thumb and forefinger) for relieving headache.

18

Stroking, Holding, and Snuggling

SOME OF THE MOST SATISFYING FORMS OF TOUCH ARE THE
simplest. There may be times when your partner is in too much discomfort, is too sensitive, or is simply too tired to tolerate the stimulation
of massage or acupressure techniques. He or she may prefer to just be
quiet together but might still welcome some form of soothing. There
may also be times when you are too tired to use other techniques but
still want to offer some kind of contact. In these circumstances, simple
stroking, holding, or snuggling can each be a welcome and comforting
form of support.

Perhaps you can remember how your parents soothed you when you
were very young. Did they lightly stroke your head or your hair? For
some people, this is reminiscent of mother's comfort in early childhood
and evokes a tangible body memory of deep relaxation and peace. That
kind of stroking actually requires close attention on the part of the giver
and naturally evokes compassionate feelings. And, of course, the recipient senses this. In a way, stroking is just as all-absorbing for the giver as
are the more formal massage techniques because you are naturally paying close attention to maintaining even contact, pressure, and direction
through the length of each stroke.

I remember one couple for whom simple stroking was especially
valuable during recovery from surgery. Sarah was recovering from a hip
replacement and had a lot of bodywide discomfort. To her, the most
wonderful thing Mark could do was to simply stroke her arm, repeatedly,
from the elbow down across the back of her hand and fingers. She described this as a divine experience because she didn't have to do anything
to respond and didn't have to be in any certain position to receive it. On
nights when she had difficulty getting to sleep, Mark would stroke her
arm this way for a few minutes, and it seemed to have an almost hypnotic
effect, as she would be able to doze off in a matter of minutes.

If stroking evokes body memories of parental soothing, so, too, do simple holding and snuggling. The most primal experience of comfort we have is that of being held close by mother. As an infant, the experience is one of being encapsulated in her arms. Being held, snuggled, or spooned by one's partner (both lying on their sides, one behind the other, with arms wrapped around him or her) is reminiscent of this protection of mother—or even of the womb.

The tactile contact with these forms of touch is obviously much greater than with manual touch such as stroking. Beyond that, however, there is also the dimension of subtle energy. Energy-based traditions of health and healing teach that we are surrounded and penetrated by a field of vital energy, and when we are holding another person close, our energy fields comingle and interpenetrate. This energetic communion is the foundation of tantric practices that seek to join energies with another in pursuit of higher spiritual states. But in the simple experiences of holding, snuggling, and spooning, you can just imagine your energy fields resting together as they occupy the same space. One practical teaching from the tantric traditions is that by synchronizing breathing with your partner—joining him or her on the in-breath and on the out-breath—you encourage this communion and harmonization of energy fields.

Many couples like the comfort of resting or even falling asleep in a spooning embrace. You can make it more comfortable with a little attention to props such as cushions, pillows, or bedding that can easily be arranged to support your heads, arms, and especially knees. This will enable you to hold any snuggle position for a longer period of time, making it a deeply relaxing and comforting experience for both partners.

PART FOUR

Simple Energy Healing
Practices

19

Energy, Intention, and Healing

OF ALL THE VARIETIES OF COMPLEMENTARY AND ALTERNA-
tive therapies, energy healing is perhaps the most intriguing and mysti-
fying. It's also fun, especially for couples. Even though it doesn't seem
to fit neatly into any of the pockets of modern science, an abundance
of evidence has established that real things happen to real people with
energy healing. Let me illustrate this with the story of Bob and Mary,
who were participants in the Caring and Cancer Project and shared the
following experience during a focus group meeting.

Mary, a fifty-five-year-old breast cancer survivor, had been having
great difficulty sleeping at night due to the hot flashes caused by her
medication—a common experience for millions of women on Tamoxifen, a form of hormone therapy to prevent recurrence of breast cancer.
One night during a hot flash, she asked Bob to try a simple energy practice we had taught in the workshop.

Bob, an engineer, was openly skeptical about whether anything good
could result from such a simple technique, and Mary wasn't expecting
much either, but she was willing to try anything. "We discovered this by
accident," she recalled, "as we were just sort of joking around with it, not
taking it seriously." To their amazement, after just two minutes, Mary's
hot flashes subsided. Ever since, they have made this a routine practice at
night at the first sign of a hot flash. Together they have gained control over
her hot flashes, and the quality of her sleep has improved dramatically.

As Mary explained, "He uses a motion of 'wiping away' with his hand,
just lightly touching the skin—or not even touching—like 'wiping away
the heat.' He'll make a circular motion to wipe it off my back and my
arms, and it's amazing how much it takes away the intensity. It's a great
relief to me because there isn't anything else at this point that the doctors will let me take to relieve those symptoms. They want to get the drug
to accumulate, and it happens that the hot flashes are one of the most
severe side effects."

What Mary and Bob have been using is a simple technique that in the tradition of Healing Touch is called *Hands-in-Motion*. As they found, it can have a tangible impact even when used very briefly. In Mary's case, it seems to control a particularly unpleasant symptom, yet the more important contribution may well be that it allows her to get quality sleep. The deepest phase of sleep, called the delta phase, is when the greatest healing takes place in the body, but disturbed sleep prevents this phase from happening. This is why disordered sleep over time can adversely influence the course of a serious illness, and good-quality sleep can turn it around.

What I find especially interesting in their story is that Bob wasn't even a believer in this method at first. Apparently, belief in the method isn't necessarily a prerequisite for it to be effective. All a person needs is an open mind and a willingness to experiment. I find this a delightful outcome in light of the simplicity, the effectiveness, and the alternative—a new and costly prescription drug that has recently been announced to counter the hot flashes caused by Tamoxifen, complete with side effects of its own.[1]

I'll describe the Hands-in-Motion technique Bob used in detail in chapter 22. First, let's take a look at the basics of energy healing.

A Universal Ability

I don't believe we'll ever completely understand how energy healing works from a scientific point of view. There will always be mystery involved because energy healing straddles two realities: the earthly world of the body, grounded in the laws of physics (the electromagnetic spectrum); and an unseen dimension beyond, from which our life energy (chi, prana, vital force) originates and to which it returns when the physical body finally wears out. But science can certainly tell us if and when it works, as we'll see later in this chapter.

Historically, there have been many approaches to working with energy for healing purposes. One of the oldest is the ancient Taoist Chinese practice of qigong, but most spiritual traditions have also embraced aspects of energy healing in one way or another. Modern times have seen the evolution of various systems, such as Therapeutic Touch, Healing Touch,

Reiki, pranic healing, SHEN Therapy, Polarity Therapy, and others in order to codify ways of working with energy. Each tradition claims its own history, training programs, and turf in the health care marketplace, but the details and differences among them don't matter nearly as much as what they all share in common. These commonalities can be summed up by two core principles. The first is that we are all beings of energy, and the second is that each of us is capable of influencing another's energy system—we are all capable of being instruments of healing. Let me elaborate.

WE ARE ALL BEINGS OF ENERGY

We each have an invisible energy system that is superimposed over, and interpenetrates with, our physical body. This energy system is the home of that mysterious force that animates us throughout life and then departs at the moment of death. That force has been called by many names: life force, vital force, life essence, chi, prana, spirit, and others. It cannot be captured or measured by technological instruments, yet it is the force that generates healing.

The many energy healing traditions share the understanding that life energy circulates through and around us continuously. Some use the Chinese concepts of the network of *acupuncture meridians* (pathways), *acupuncture points* (tiny "way stations" along the meridians), and *dantiens* (energy centers on the body). Some use Indian concepts that are roughly parallel, called the *nadis, marma points,* and *chakras.* All conceive of our energy system as reaching out into multiple layers of energy fields that surround our bodies like layers of an onion extending several inches out from the surface.

Whatever the vocabulary, the common understanding is that our physical body and our energy system are intertwined. Good health is an expression of balanced and harmonious circulation of energy, and ill health is an expression of disharmony, imbalance, or blockages to the circulation of energy. Thus, all energy healing traditions focus their efforts on restoring the proper harmony and balanced circulation of energy.

There is recent scientific evidence to confirm these principles. Our meridians have been found to emit light, which can be seen with infrared photography,[2] and researchers have even found evidence that illness is associated with emission of less light from the meridians.[3] The light comes from ions flowing along "ionic streambeds" in the interstitial layer of tissue just beneath the surface of our skin, and these pathways correspond with the geography of the meridians recognized for thousands of years.[4] These flowing streams of ions are not our life energy itself but are regarded as a parallel *electromagnetic effect* and *indicator* of the flow of life energy. The specific points along the meridians have also been studied; they have much higher electrical conductivity and higher amplitude of the electric current wave than do other points on our body.[5]

The existence of the chakras has been supported by studies using electrodes directly on the surface of the skin[6] as well as some distance away from the body.[7] Photons (units of light) are emitted from the locations of the chakras, and researchers have found that by concentrating the mind on a certain chakra, people can dramatically increase the number of photons being emitted.[8] As with the acupuncture points and meridians, what can be measured in these cases is not life energy itself but may be considered secondary effects of the circulation of our life energy—in a sense, its *imprint* in the physical domain.

With so much going on in the body energetically, it's easy to imagine how all of these forces can combine to create an energy *field* that radiates several inches beyond the surface of the skin, called the "aura" or "biofield." Many energy healing practices work "off the body" in this surrounding field; indeed, in many of studies I'll be noting later, healing effects occurred with no physical contact whatsoever.

WE ARE ALL CAPABLE OF BEING INSTRUMENTS OF HEALING

By just being *present*, using *mental intention*, and *using your hands in simple ways*, you can be an instrument of healing.

The starting point for all this is *presence*. Being fully present means centering yourself—clearing your mind of distracting thoughts or anxieties, so that your awareness is fully available to be focused on what is happening here and now. It requires that you occupy a state of concentration and nondistractibility that may be described as "sustained attention." This quality of presence is key to being able to work with energy. Simple centering exercises or meditations (as described in the chapters to follow) are usually recommended to establish presence and sustained attention.[9]

Once you are fully present, your mental *intention* (also called *intentionality*) is essential for energy healing to happen. Intention is, of course, a fuzzy concept, and no one can really say in detail how it works. Marilyn Schlitz, director of research at the Institute of Noetic Sciences, has defined intentionality as involving "the projection of awareness, with purpose and efficacy, toward some object or outcome."[10]

You need only contemplate the act of lifting your finger right now to experience the incredible mystery of intention. You can lift your finger when you intend to, but why, really, does it move? You might say that your brain is sending a neural impulse to the muscles to contract in a certain way, but what is the true origin of that impulse?

A similar mystery surrounds the relationship between intention and energy; an old saying in Chinese medicine attempts to capture the relationship this way: "Where the mind goes, the chi follows." As you'll see in the studies mentioned below, experiments have been conducted comparing authentic energy healing techniques with "sham," or fake, treatments in which a treater uses his or her hands in a similar way but is instructed to think about something else (such as counting backward from one hundred by threes). Several such studies have confirmed the idea that intention is the key to the effects of energy healing.

Intention may be of two kinds, and it's not clear that either is superior to the other. It may be directive, such as the intention for energy to flow easily and freely between your hands along a certain pathway in the recipient's body, or for energy to disperse from an area where it has been congested. You might use visualization or specific hand movements through the person's energy field to encourage this to happen, as Bob did with Mary.

It may also be nondirective, in the form of simple intentions like "May the highest good prevail," "Thy will be done," or "May I be an instrument of Thy peace." These intentions work well, too. Many people prefer them because they invoke participation of Higher Intelligence or Spirit to do what is truly needed, which may be beyond our understanding. This affirms a sense of humility and helps to keep one's ego at bay in deference to the great mystery that healing is and from where it comes. This kind of intention may, of course, be joined with a directive one, as in the intention for energy to move through an area "if it is Thy will," always retaining the ultimate focus on the highest good.

Finally, your *hands* are particularly versatile tools because they can sense, send, and move energy. Other forms of contact with another person can influence his or her energy as well—in fact, just being in the person's energy field a few inches away without physically touching can have an impact. But your hands are the main tools of energy healing—perhaps because they are extensions of your heart, your body's strongest energy center. You can use your hands to balance the flow of energy between two points, stimulate the flow through a certain area, clear out blockages to the flow of energy, soothe and even out the energy field, direct energy into a target area, and many other uses.

A Look at the Evidence

There have been literally hundreds of studies on the many forms of energy healing testifying to benefits for all kinds of health conditions. Historically, they have been criticized as lacking research designs that could accurately evaluate the effects, but recent years have seen a real jump in the quality of studies, especially as the National Institutes of Health has begun funding work in this area.

There are now many studies that meet the scientific gold standard of the randomized controlled trial. The best-designed ones have been done with the most widely practiced methods—mainly Therapeutic Touch and, to lesser degrees, Healing Touch and Reiki. Other methods have been studied, but these three have been looked at most closely by mainstream researchers. Collectively, these studies do a good job of representing what is possible with energy healing.

Since there haven't been any head-to-head comparisons, there is no evidence that one form of energy healing is superior to any other. So let me reiterate what I consider to be a very important point: in the big picture, the common principles and common effects across all forms are much more important than any subtle differences of technique among them (though some advocates of specific individual methods might disagree with this statement). The research shows that your presence and the intentionality that you bring to the experience are the real keys to having a beneficial effect for another. For this reason, and for ease of understanding, in the brief research review to follow, I will refer to all the methods as simply "energy healing," or EH for short.[11]

GENERAL EFFECTS

Regardless of a person's main symptom or problem, energy healing seems to affect the whole person on all levels simultaneously. This makes sense if you think about how energy circulates continuously throughout the whole person and is not compartmentalized or localized to just one area. It's a little like treating a person's blood—wherever you treat it, it's going to have effects bodywide.

One of the most obvious and common effects of energy healing is that it encourages relaxation. In fact, many researchers believe that the relaxation response might be the main reason for its benefits. The relaxation response is a physiological change in which your heart rate, blood pressure, and tension decrease, while relaxation, peace of mind, and immune functioning increase. This argument gains support from a comparison of the results of studies in energy healing with studies in meditation, relaxation training, and imagery. All seem to lead to this similar pattern of benefits for both body and mind. This may be the main reason why energy therapies are so universally enjoyed regardless of the particular ailment.

Confirmation of the link to relaxation was found in a recent Scottish study in which researchers randomly assigned forty-five healthy people to either an authentic EH session, a simple rest period, or a sham EH session by someone who mimicked the movements of an energy healer but without the use of positive intention. In the group receiving the authentic treatment, both heart rate and blood pressure—major indicators of relaxation—were significantly reduced compared to the other two groups.[12] An earlier study looked at psychological effects of EH in forty-one healthy females over time. Women who received a three-session series showed significant reductions on psychological scales measuring tension, confusion, and anxiety and a significant increase in vigor compared to their counterparts who did not receive the series.[13]

Results like these are commonplace in studies of meditation and relaxation techniques. It's pretty clear from both research and practical experience that deep relaxation is an important and beneficial by-product of energy healing.

PAIN

One of the strongest areas of research for energy healing is in pain reduction. This makes sense when you think of pain as signifying a blockage or an impairment of energy flow through the body. Headache pain seems to respond particularly well. For example, in one study, sixty patients with tension headache were assigned to either authentic EH or a sham version in which the practitioner used identical hand movements but used a mental distraction technique in place of the healing intention. Four hours later, the patients in the authentic treatment group had significantly greater reductions in pain levels than the other subjects.[14]

Arthritis also responds well. In one study, eighty-two elderly adults with arthritis received either a weekly session of EH, a weekly session of relaxation training, or usual care only for six weeks. Pain, tension, mood, and satisfaction improved after both EH and progressive muscle relaxation. Hand function improved after EH; walking and bending improved after progressive muscle relaxation, but overall functional ability was significantly better for the EH group.[15]

And in a study of osteoarthritis of the knee, twenty-five patients were assigned to either authentic EH, mock EH (identical hand movements conducted by an untrained person), or usual care only, weekly for six weeks. In the EH group, severity of pain was significantly reduced, and general activity level was improved.[16]

Energy healing is used for relief by many sufferers of fibromyalgia, which can bring bodywide pain. A small study evaluated the effects of an EH technique in six women with fibromyalgia and found significant reductions in pain as well as overall improvements in their quality of life.[17]

The use of EH services in hospitals for postoperative pain is becoming very common. One study randomly assigned 108 postoperative patients to five minutes of authentic EH, sham EH, or standard pain medication. While the medication was more effective than EH at reducing pain, those who received EH waited significantly longer before asking for pain medication than those who received the sham treatment.[18] In another hospital-based study, seriously ill patients in critical care were found to have enhanced relaxation and sleep with the help of EH.[19]

Burn victims have been of special interest to energy healing researchers because the pain is so hard to treat. In an important study that demonstrated the value of off-body energy healing, researchers assigned ninety-nine adult burn patients to five treatments over six days of either authentic EH or sham EH (identical hand movements conducted by an untrained person who also practiced a mental distraction technique). Compared to the sham controls, authentic EH patients had significantly greater reductions in pain and lower anxiety levels.[20]

EFFECTS ON MOOD

Many studies have explored the effects of EH on mood, particularly anxiety and depression—either by themselves or as they accompany a medical illness. In one, forty-six people suffering from depression were randomly assigned to receive hands-on EH, sham EH (without the intention), or distant healing (see part 5). Those receiving either authentic EH or distant healing had significant improvements in measures of psychological distress compared to the sham group.[21] Another study assigned sixty patients in a cardiovascular care unit to a single treatment of EH or a sham version (minus the healing intention). A 17 percent drop in anxiety scores was found after the authentic treatment.[22] EH has also been shown to reduce anxiety in such diverse groups as the institutionalized elderly[23] and pregnant women who are undergoing treatment for chemical dependency.[24]

CANCER

Energy healing is used a great deal in cancer support programs to help patients cope with pain and treatment side effects. The general effects noted above are seen in cancer of all types and stages.

In terms of more specific studies, one study randomly assigned ten terminal cancer patients to three sessions of EH and ten other patients to simply rest for an equivalent time period. Those receiving the treatment achieved significantly better scores on well-being and symptoms of discomfort.[25] Energy healing has also been studied in women undergoing radiation therapy for cancer, with such benefits as reductions in cancer-related fatigue and improvements in ratings of overall quality of life.[26] In other work, it has been found to improve pain control and quality of life in advanced cancer patients.[27]

And in a large study done at the University of Minnesota with 230 cancer patients receiving chemotherapy, researchers compared both massage and EH to the simple presence of a caring nurse or standard care with no special healing activity. Both EH and massage lowered blood pressure, respiratory rate, pain, heart rate, and mood disturbance, all indicators of the relaxation response. In addition, EH reduced fatigue, a major symptom that compromises quality of life in chemotherapy patients.[28]

EFFECTS ON BRAIN FUNCTIONING

One of the more mysterious aspects of energy healing is its potential to influence brain functioning. This is of growing interest given the rapidly increasing population of elderly people. The brain/mind relationship is, of course, extremely complex, and a variety of avenues have been used in the name of improving a person's mental functioning, from drugs to psychotherapy.

According to two recent studies in Alzheimer's dementia, energy healing may be a new source of hope for brain-related disorders associated with aging. In one, researchers were interested in reducing troubling behavioral symptoms such as restlessness, escaping restraints, searching and wandering, tapping and banging, pacing and walking, and vocalization in fifty-seven elderly nursing home residents with dementia. Those who received treatment with EH for just five to seven minutes a day, twice a day for three days, showed significant reductions in symptoms compared to residents who received a sham version of the technique.[29] Further, a study with patients in the advanced stages of Alzheimer's dementia found that those who received five sessions of EH had significantly lower levels of agitation and irritability than a comparison group receiving five sessions of simple presence by a caregiver.[30]

There are also numerous case reports of dementia or stroke benefiting from energy healing. I once knew a terminal cancer patient who had had a stroke that rendered him unable to speak. During his last week of life, his children arranged for a couple of EH treatments just to help him be comfortable. Amazingly, after each treatment, he regained his ability to speak for about two hours, after which it would slowly fade away again. This was an invaluable opportunity for him to communicate with his loved ones during his final days and was healing for all. I have heard other similar reports concerning stroke and energy healing. It appears that the neurological system may be particularly responsive to subtle energetic influences.

In summary, the studies noted above are but recent highlights in a huge body of work. The evidence indicates that energy healing can have benefits for pain in a wide variety of conditions, as well as mood, overall functioning, and quality of life in chronic conditions such as cancer, arthritis, or fibromyalgia. We don't know how much the benefits are due to generalized effects such as the relaxation response as opposed to more detailed effects induced by specific intentions or techniques of the practitioner. The studies do, however, affirm the critical role of intention on the part of the practitioner.

The research in this field has generally been done using professionally trained practitioners. However, one of the greatest myths about energy healing is that it requires special training and can only be done by professionals. In reality, the ability to be fully present and use intention are the key ingredients; the techniques of how you use your hands *give form to the expression* of intention, but they are not the most important factor. The techniques certainly don't need to be done perfectly in order to have positive effects. This was our message to the participants in the Caring and Cancer and Elder Healer projects, and the successes of the participants have shown it to be true.

The following chapters offer several energy techniques you can experiment with. They are safe and have no history of adverse effects, so you can relax as you explore them. As long as you stay true to being present and focused on your intention, you can't go wrong. Keep the dialogue with your partner open and have fun.

20

Balancing Energy

POLARITY THERAPY IS A TRADITION OF HANDS-ON HEALING based on the principle that energy flows through the body along predict-able pathways. It holds that illness or symptoms result when the flow is impaired or out of balance and that the proper flow can be reestablished by the giver's placing his or her hands at strategic points (which serve as opposite poles relative to each other) on the recipient's body. This tradi-tion also extends the metaphor of positive and negative polarities into other aspects of the person's life, such as nutrition and exercise, all in the service of maintaining the proper circulation of energy through the body/mind system.

Polarity Therapy has not been as widely studied as some other forms of energy healing, but research has recently been sponsored by the Na-tional Institutes of Health to explore its effects on stress reduction and quality of life in caregivers. Also, there is some evidence that it may help reduce fatigue in people undergoing radiation therapy.[1] The benefits are most likely broad-spectrum, in the sense that stress reduction and relaxation naturally help reduce all kinds of symptoms. You can use the technique below with any health condition, and your partner will enjoy its pleasant effects.

The Five-Pointed Star

The Five-Pointed Star is a simple technique of Polarity Therapy that is designed to balance your partner's energy and encourage peace and relaxation. It is done with your partner lying on his or her back and you standing or seated at the right. Imagine a five-pointed star overlaying your partner's body: one point just inside each hip bone (over the psoas muscle, referred to as the "hip point"), one on the front of each shoulder, and one at the base of the throat (the "throat center").

Begin by centering yourself. Take a few moments to breathe deeply and access a state of compassionate intention for your partner's highest good.

1. Now, using very light touch with just your fingertips, reach across to your partner's left hip point with your right fingertips, and place your left fingertips lightly at the throat point. Imagine a straight line of energy connecting these two points. Be careful to keep the touch very light. Hold these contacts until you sense a pulsation coming up under your fingertips and beating harmoniously and at the same rate under the fingertips of each hand.

2. Keeping your left fingertips where they are, move your right fingertips to the right hip point. Again, visualize a line of energy passing through the diaphragm connecting these two points. Take your time and continue to breathe in a relaxed way. Hold these positions until you again sense a slight pulsation under the fingertips of each hand and you sense that the line has come into balance.

3. Keeping your right fingertips where they are, move your left hand to the left shoulder point, creating a diagonal through the diaphragm to the right hip point. Visualize a line of energy moving across the center of the body through the diaphragm to connect these two points.

4. Finally, move your left hand to the right shoulder and your right hand to the left hip point, again visualizing a diagonal line of energy connecting these points.

Throughout this process, let your movements be very slow and gentle, and remember to breathe so you can be as relaxed and present as possible. When finished, you may want to hold your partner's feet for grounding.

If you want to learn more about energy balancing or study Polarity Therapy, visit the Web site of the American Polarity Therapy Association.[2]

21

Clearing the Field

CLEARING THE FIELD IS AN OFF-BODY MANUAL TECHNIQUE in which you move your hands down the entire length of your partner's energy field from head to toe in a gentle, broad sweeping or brushing motion. Sometimes called clearing, unruffling, smoothing, magnetic passes, or stroking the cat, the purpose is to clear the person's energy field of loose congestion, harmonizing the flow of vital energy throughout the system. This is a core element of both the Therapeutic Touch and Healing Touch traditions and was used in both the Caring and Cancer Project and the Elder Healer Project.

The image of stroking a cat's fur is very apt in that a cat's fur grows in one direction, from head to toe. If there are areas where it is matted, mussed up or disorganized, grooming or stroking it will realign the hairs and the coat returns to its original smooth and neat state, with all the hairs flowing together again in an uninterrupted, smooth, and unified system. This is a good metaphor for clearing and smoothing a person's energy field.

Steps for Clearing the Field

WASH YOUR HANDS

Before beginning you may want to wash your hands to feel clean and confident that you're not introducing any unwanted energy into your partner's energy field.

GET PERMISSION

Be sure you have your partner's permission to work. Ask him or her to describe any symptoms or problem areas for you to be aware of.

GET COMFORTABLE

Make sure both of you are in a comfortable position. Your partner may be sitting upright or lying down. You can be standing or sitting next to your partner, but make sure you that your posture is not a strain for you, as this will create tension in your body and interfere with your ability to be completely present.

CENTER YOURSELF

As with all other healing techniques, it's a good idea to begin with a few moments of centering to become fully present. Close your eyes, bring your attention to your breath, and focus on following your breath for a few moments. Use the breath to help you let go of any mental distractions. Breathe in a series of full, satisfying breaths. On each out-breath, imagine exhaling any distracting thoughts and releasing any expectations or pressures for performance or outcomes of this experience. Remember that your hands are extensions of your heart. Focus on the main intention to be a peaceful and healing presence for your mate and "Thy will be done." Stay with this until you have reached a feeling of centeredness, calm, and peace.

MAKE SLOW SWEEPS DOWN THE FIELD

Holding your hands a few inches above your partner's body with palms facing down, start at the head and move your hands continuously and slowly down the length of the body through the field. Make several slow sweeps down the length of the body, from the head down the sides and from the head down over the middle. You may use as many as fifteen one-minute cycles down each side of the body. There is no set number of times or length of time; just do what feels right to you.

NOTICE DIFFERENCES

As you make sweeps down the field, you may notice subtle differences from one area to the next, such as gradations of temperature, a sensation of heaviness or thickness, lightness or thinness, and so forth. If you don't notice any differences as you move though the field, don't worry, this is not a problem. It may be that there are none to notice, or it may be that with more practice, you might begin to notice more.

The use of the clearing motions may in itself change these sensations without your focusing on them directly. In the Hands-in-Motion technique (chapter 22), you will work with a localized area to try to even those differences out, but during simple clearing, you're not attempting to work in a localized area. Again, if no differences are apparent to you, don't be concerned.

GROUND YOUR PARTNER

When you finish, if you are not going to move on to other techniques, ground the person by holding his or her feet for a few moments.

COMPLETE THE PROCESS

Talk with your partner about what each of you experienced. Then just sit quietly together for a few moments before moving on to other activities. You may want to wash your hands afterward to cleanse them of any unwanted energy and feel refreshed.

22

Local Clearing

YOU CAN SOMETIMES HAVE AN IMPACT ON A LOCAL AREA OF pain or discomfort such as a strain, sprain, muscle ache, headache, or joint pain by moving your hands through the energy field above it for a targeted local clearing effect. You can use this over regions of the body such as low back, head, neck, shoulders, knees, or any other specific areas. Use can be brief—your partner may notice benefits within just a few moments of using the method by itself. It may also be used as part of a longer treatment session in combination with other methods. This concept is used in a variety of healing traditions; in the Healing Touch program it is referred to simply as Hands-in-Motion.

This method is based on the simple understanding that pain or dysfunction in an area of the body is mirrored by disturbance in the energy field over and around that area. With Hands-in-Motion, your intention is to break up congestion in the energy field and restore the smooth flow and circulation of energy through the particular region where the person is experiencing the problem. As Mary and Bob showed in chapter 19, encouraging the flow of energy through Mary's back and arms was enough to significantly diminish her hot flashes.

Steps for Local Clearing

If you haven't already done so, begin with the steps outlined in chapter 21 for Clearing the Field (washing your hands, getting permission to work, getting comfortable, and centering yourself). Then ask the recipient to describe the symptom or problem and where it is located.

EXPLORATION

When ready, very slowly, gently, and respectfully enter the person's energy field with your hands palms-down two to five inches above the skin but a few inches *away* from the problem area. This will enable you to get a sense of how the field seems to feel outside the problem area. Move your hands slowly through the surrounding area two to five inches above the skin and then gradually over the problem area. Move your hands around to see if you might notice subtle gradations of temperature between the surrounding areas and the problem area. You might also see if you can notice other subtle sensations with your hands, such as a feeling of thickness or heaviness or lightness in the field as you move from one area to another.

If you do notice any sensations of differentness from one area to another, this may help you get a sense of where to concentrate your work. But don't worry if you don't notice any differences—they may not be noticeable, or you may simply begin to notice them with more practice. If you don't notice differences, then just rely on your partner's description of where the problem is.

LOCAL CLEARING

Now begin a stroking motion through and over the area of concern—again, two to five inches above the skin. Simply move your hands slowly and deliberately in a smooth stroking movement as if you were stroking a cat in the direction of the fur. Imagine that the fur has been ruffled or mussed up and you are smoothing it and restoring the alignment of all the hairs. You could also imagine using your fingers like a comb, bending them slightly as if you were running them through the fur to help straighten and reorganize it.

Continue to breathe and maintain a sense of centeredness in your breath, as you slowly and gently move your hands through the person's energy field over the target area. All movements should be slow and relaxed, not fast or jerky.

You may do this for just a minute or two, or you may want to continue longer, perhaps five or ten minutes; it's up to the two of you. You and your partner can talk during this process about what sensations each of you is feeling. Either of you can let the other know when you feel finished.

FINISHING UP

If you are not going to move on to other techniques, do the grounding and completion steps, as outlined at the end of chapter 21 ("Clearing the Field").

᾽ ᾽ ᾽

There are many possible variations on this technique, but the common elements are described above. And, of course, you can use it in conjunction with clearing or other techniques before or after. If you'd like to learn more, a good resource is Dorothea Hover-Kramer's *Healing Touch: A Guidebook for Practitioners*, second edition (Delmar, 2002).

23

Chakra Connection

THE CHAKRAS ARE ENERGY CENTERS THAT FUNCTION LIKE way stations or gateways for the flow of energy through the entire energy system within and around the body. Minor chakras are located in the joints, and major chakras are located generally up the centerline of the body.

The Chakra Connection is a basic full-body balancing technique to encourage the flow of energy from chakra to chakra by connecting the major and minor chakras. The technique was developed and defined by W. Brugh Joy, MD, in his book *Joy's Way*.[1]

In this method, you use your hands to connect, open, and balance the energy centers and to enhance the flow of energy through your partner's body. It can be done on yourself or with two people doing it on a third person. The technique requires activation of the energy in your hands in order to facilitate energy movement through the recipient's body.

The sequence of steps is described below. It can be done with the recipient either lying down or seated. Begin on the person's right side and follow the sequence as shown.

Energy healing is not an exact science, and much of what you do will be influenced by your intuitive sense of what you are feeling. Generally, however, your hand positions are held in place for approximately one minute or until you can feel a sensation of active energy flow between your hands. Move up the body from the feet to the head.

When you do move your hands from one pair of positions to the next, move them one at a time so that one hand is always in contact with your partner.

Steps for the Chakra Connection

If you haven't already done so, begin with the steps outlined in chapter 21 for Clearing the Field (washing your hands, getting permission to work, getting comfortable, and centering yourself).

For the Chakra Connection, your partner can be lying on his or her back with you standing along the right side of the body. Alternatively, this technique can be used with the person sitting in a chair, in which case you will need to sit or kneel alongside in order to reach the holding positions. Once you are centered and ready to make contact, follow these steps.

1. Place your lower (right) hand on the recipient's right ankle and your upper (left) hand on his or her right knee. Then move gradually up to each of the following pairs of positions.
2. The right knee and hip.
3. The left ankle and knee. (Note: You can stay standing where you are and reach across so your right hand is on the left ankle and your left hand is on the left knee. However, if this is uncomfortable, you can walk around to the left side of the body, and your left hand becomes the lower hand. If you do walk to the other side, keep one hand in contact with your partner as you move.)
4. Left knee and hip.
5. Both hips.
6. Root and sacral chakras. The root chakra opens under the pelvis at the perineum between the legs. Rather than placing your hand on it directly you can hold you hand in the air slightly above and part way down the thighs toward the knees, with your palm angled toward the perineum. The sacrum chakra is situated a couple of inches below the navel.
7. Sacrum and solar plexus chakras. The solar plexus chakra is a couple of inches below the hollow at the base of the sternum (chest bone).
8. Solar plexus and spleen. The spleen chakra is adjacent to the solar plexus in the left side of the abdomen and slightly lower, just beneath the middle of the bottom rib.
9. Solar plexus and heart chakra. The heart chakra is at the center of the chest. For women you can just use your fingertips on the breastbone or hold your hand above the body.
10. Heart chakra and high heart. The high heart is behind the upper portion of the breast bone.
11. Right wrist and elbow.

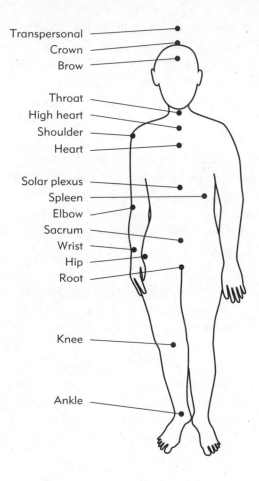

Transpersonal
Crown
Brow

Throat
High heart
Shoulder
Heart

Solar plexus
Spleen
Elbow
Sacrum
Wrist
Hip
Root

Knee

Ankle

12. Right elbow and shoulder.

13. Left wrist and elbow.

14. Left elbow and shoulder.

15. Both shoulders. You can do this either reaching across to the far shoulder, or standing at the head to reach both shoulders more comfortably.

16. High heart and throat chakra. For the throat chakra, rest the thumb edge of your upper hand on the collarbone with your elbow raised and your palm angled toward the throat, so your hand is not directly on the throat.

17. Throat chakra and brow chakra. Rest the little finger–edge of your lower hand on the collar bone with the palm angled toward

the throat. The brow chakra is right between the eyebrows and slightly above.

18. Brow chakra and crown chakra. The crown chakra is at the top of the head.

19. Crown chakra and transpersonal point. Picture the centerline of the body continuing straight out beyond the crown chakra. The transpersonal point is visualized about eight to ten inches out beyond the crown along that line. To hold these two points you have to turn both palms outward as though you are parting a pair of curtains. Now place the lower palm directly on the crown, and move the upper palm straight out about eight to ten inches, facing outward.

Finishing up: If you are not going to move on to other techniques, do the grounding and completion steps, as outlined at the end of chapter 21 ("Clearing the Field").

24

Zeroing In

MANY TRADITIONS TEACH THAT A HEALER CAN INTENSELY zero in on an area of pain in a recipient and direct energy into it to break up a local pattern of stuck or blocked energy. In Chinese tradition this is referred to as a form of "external" qigong (with energy being sent in from outside). The Healing Touch tradition teaches a form of this called Laser Beam, an off-body technique in which you put your thumb and two fingers of one hand together with the intention to direct a focused, penetrating beam of energy into a local area. Common targets include arthritic joints, joint injuries, fractured bones, tendonitis, sprains, or strains. This technique was taught in the Elder Healer Project and many participants reported surprising effects from it, including one who reported that it alleviated the pain from her long-standing interstitial cystitis that had not responded to medication.

Here are the instructions:

1. On one hand, hold your thumb and your first and second fingers together, and with your mental intention, direct energy from the palm chakra down through the tips of your fingers and thumb.
2. Imagine a beam of light extending out from the tips of your fingers and thumb that is directed into the local area of the recipient's body.
3. Place your other hand behind the body part you are working on. See if you can feel the beam of energy come through into that hand's palm. Some people feel nothing, and some feel a subtle sensation of heat or tingling in the receiving hand.
4. Move your sending hand in any direction in a twirling or corkscrew pattern with the fingers pointed toward the area. Keep the hand moving continuously for a few seconds. Imagine you are stirring up the energy field in the area of pain, loosening up any blockage so that energy can flow through easily again.

25

Laying On of Hands

THE TERM *LAYING ON OF HANDS* IS A FASCINATING EXPRESSION. It implies that simply resting one's hands on another can make something good happen. Clearly, whatever happens is not a result of manipulation or technique, so that leaves energy and intention. By resting your hands on your partner, you are indeed making energetic contact—in effect, joining your partner to make one energy system. Then, by focusing on compassionate intention for your partner's highest good, you set your ego aside and make yourself a doorway through which the intelligence of the universe can send whatever it wants to send for the benefit of your partner. ht

This is perhaps the most basic expression of energy healing. It is too simple for dogmatic systems to be built up around it, or for judgments of technique as right or wrong. It is purely a matter of opening yourself up to be as clean and clear a channel of goodness for your partner as you can.

Below are a couple of simple examples of how you can use laying on of hands with your partner to help encourage states of calm, peace, and relaxation.

Sitting in Peace

Have your partner sit in front of you in a chair with his or her back to you, with you sitting or standing behind. (Make sure you are comfortable.) Center yourself first with a few deep breaths and focus on the intention that the intelligence of the universe come through you and your hands to do whatever is needed for your partner's highest good. Now rest your hands on your partner's trapezius muscles—the area of tension that most people have between their neck and shoulder on either side. Just lightly rest your hands there and remember the intention. Be aware that the intention is not for you to "do" anything other than just be present but rather for you to simply be an instrument through which loving energy can pass into your partner, melting any tension in the entire body and rebalancing the circulation of energy and relaxing the muscles. Just hold this position until you feel as if your purpose has been fulfilled.

Be aware that your partner may not notice anything at all during this exercise but may discover later that he or she is more relaxed. You may also notice that you benefit as well in terms of greater relaxation, peace, or energy.

Going with the Flow

Have your partner lie down on his or her back with you seated at the side. Center yourself first with a few deep breaths and focus on the intention that the intelligence of the universe come through you and your hands to do whatever is needed for your partner's highest good.

Now cradle your partner's head in one hand by sliding your hand under the base of the skull and holding the head in a position that is comfortable for the neck, where your partner feels supported. Slide your other hand underneath his or her body at the sacrum (the bone at the base of the spine just above the tailbone, opposite the pubic bone). The idea is to support the two areas with your hands in a very gentle way, as you would hold a baby.

It may be important to have your arms supported on the mattress or cushion so you don't transmit any tension of your own through your hands and so that you can enjoy the relaxation, too.

These two points represent opposite ends of the main energy channel that flows up through the center of the body, known as the *shushumna* in yogic tradition or the cranial-sacral system in craniosacral therapy. By holding these positions, you are encouraging the free and unimpeded flow of energy through this channel, which can then have a relaxing and enlivening effect for your partner.

26

A Family Way

GWEN (THIRTY-FOUR) HAS POLYARTHRITIS, WHICH MAINLY manifests as swollen elbows and knees. The inflammation migrates around her body intermittently but consistently seems to settle most in her left knee. She can't get comfortable with it and always has a hard time getting to sleep and sleeping through the night, as the pain frequently wakes her up. She has taken a variety of conventional medications to control the pain and inflammation and has tried antidepressants but went off them due to the side effects. I had seen her about four times individually to work on some mind-body techniques for coping with the pain and then suggested a family meeting to teach her husband, George (thirty-six), and her children, Rosalie (three) and Johnny (seven), some simple techniques of Healing Touch they could experiment with at home.

When the family arrived, we first talked with the children about times they have been hurt and what they did. Rosalie recalled falling down and hurting both knees, and how her mother got a Band-Aid and held her to make her feel better. Johnny spoke of falling off of a scooter going down a hill and skinning both knees and elbows, and how his friends responded by getting a washcloth and warm water and soap to clean his wounds. We made the point that it feels good to have attention from others who care when you are hurting. I then asked the kids if they were aware of mom's sore knee, and they both said they were. I explained that just as she does things to help them feel better when they are hurting, they can do things to help her feel better when her knee is hurting.

We then moved a massage table into the center of the room and Gwen lay down on her back. I stood at the left shoulder, Rosalie stood on a chair at the right shoulder, Johnny stood at the left knee, and George at the right knee. I explained that what we were going to do was send love through our hands into her body. I then asked them to rub their hands together to feel the warmth and to imagine this was love in their hands. I asked them to imagine sending the love from their hands into their mother's body. Next I had them very gently and slowly rest their hands on her joints using the Chakra Connection positions, with each person holding two joints (ankle-knee and shoulder-wrist on each side). I coached them to imagine the love flowing between their hands and to imagine their favorite color flowing between their hands representing that love. I also suggested the image of the love flowing from their heart down their arms through their hands into their mother's body.

Both children were surprisingly compliant, not something commonly seen in family meetings with children that age. Whereas prior to the exercise they were fidgeting and moving about the room, they became captivated by the process as the four of us stayed with it for about twenty minutes. I gave them lots of reinforcement and congratulations as we went along, and both remained silent as they appeared mystified by the process.

We moved around among the various joint combinations (sole-knee; ankle-hip; wrist-shoulder, elbow-shoulder) used in the Chakra Connection, but for simplicity we concentrated on the joints and did not work with the main chakras directly. The primary instruction to George and the children was to continue breathing and imagining the love flowing between their hands. I reminded them several times that when thoughts come into their minds, they can just bring their attention back to the love between their hands and that they don't need to do anything else.

Next we did simple holding positions, with hands above and below each joint (each knee, each elbow) to imagine concentrating the love in that specific joint. Each person imagined his or her own favorite color flowing between the two hands representing his or her love—pink for Rosalie, red for Johnny, and blue-purple for George.

This was followed by "stroking the cat," a perfect metaphorical name for the technique of clearing or unruffling used in touch therapy, as the children had two cats at home. We imagined slowly stroking their fur from head to toe, a couple of inches above Gwen's body. Finally we closed with George and the children holding Gwen's feet with their hands for grounding.

Gwen was tearful and hugged everyone individually, remarking about how loved she felt. I encouraged them to practice a few minutes whenever they can, with an optimal time of fifteen to twenty minutes, but emphasized that even five minutes could be beneficial.

A week later, I saw Gwen alone. She reported that when they got home from the prior session, Johnny had been eager to show his friend how to do Healing Touch and also showed his friend's mother. Both Johnny and Rosalie practiced on Gwen several time since as well. Then she told me that the night before, for the first time since our last meeting, she asked George if he would try the Healing Touch on her knee. He worked on her left leg and left arm, placing his hands on and around the joints in the various sequences. He ended with the brushing movements through her energy field, as we had practiced as a family, and then held her feet at the end. She stated that the pain went away and she was able to sleep through the whole night with no problem. Also, she noticed that there had been almost no pain during the day.

I recommended that she ask her children and husband for this kind of support regularly and see if it contributes to improved sleep quality on a consistent basis. If it does, this could have global benefits for her condition. She is now considering using the techniques with George, who suffers from insomnia.

PART FIVE

Distant Healing

27

Never Beyond Reach

ONE OF THE MOST COMMON WAYS WE ALL FUNCTION AS HEAL-
ers, perhaps even without realizing it, is through our private prayers and
mental intentions. Larry Dossey, MD, author of *Reinventing Medicine,*
has made a compelling argument that prayer and related "distant healing" practices that project positive intentionality across distance are part
of a new "nonlocal medicine" that is the next great step beyond mind-
body medicine.[1]

There is no question psychological comfort and tangible forms of day-
to-day support can make a big difference in the stress level of someone
living with a serious illness, reducing symptoms and possibly even prolonging life. But what if you could—in the words of Phil from the introduction—"reach into" your partner's body and influence healing from
within? The prospect of being able to exert such influence from a distance could indeed be a source of encouragement and empowerment.

How Might Distant Healing Be Possible?

There are three broad points of view on how distant healing might occur.
One uses the logic of religion, which holds that it occurs through inter-
cession by a higher power beyond our understanding. All the world's
religions regard prayer as a means by which we can ask God, Spirit, or
some other entity that is beyond us to intervene on behalf of another.
Whether that entity actually listens to us, and how it regards our requests, is a theological question, but in this perspective it is that higher
power that does the work or performs the miracle.

The second uses the logic of mysticism, which holds that we are all
connected through an unseen dimension of reality, and we can personally wield influence for the healing of another person through that unseen connection. This idea can open the door for our ego to get involved,
either through an inflated perception of our own power or through

feelings of failure and despair if our expected results do not materialize. Nevertheless, it is possible to keep one's ego tucked in and consider that the ability to influence others through an unseen dimension may be a natural birthright we all share, something that some of us simply may have developed more than others.

A third possibility is integrative, considering distant healing as a co-creative activity, with you, a higher intelligence, and the recipient all working together, with the cooperation of all three in place in order for good things to happen. This perspective straddles the boundaries of religion, mysticism, and science. It allows that there will always be an element of mystery as to how and why distant influence might occur. But we might be able to borrow some insights from the world of physics to help understand how such a cocreative process might unfold.

QUANTUM ENTANGLEMENT

One of the most helpful concepts I've found for understanding the possibility of distant healing is "quantum entanglement." This is a rather intriguing idea borrowed from the field of quantum physics to explain how two people in an intimate relationship may, over time, develop a level of connectedness and mutual influence that transcends time and space.

Through its theory of quantum mechanics, modern physics explains how two subatomic particles that have been in close proximity to each other maintain a relationship of reciprocal influence on each other across unlimited distance when separated—a phenomenon called "nonlocal connectedness." This idea is captured in Bell's theorem and is based on the observation that two subatomic particles that were once in contact with each other show qualities of enduring connectedness after they have been shot through a photon gun and become well separated in space. Specifically, when the spin of one changes, the spin of the other changes—simultaneously and to the same degree. The two particles retain some mysterious kind of reciprocal nonlocal connectedness across distance.

The key insight that Bell's theorem offers is that a change in one particle is reflected in the other *simultaneously*, without the time delay required for the transmittal of a signal over the distance between them. Thus, there appears to be a *correlational* relationship between the two particles, as if they are two aspects of one unified whole, rather than a *causal* relationship, in which one entity influences what happens in the other.

Einstein was fascinated with nonlocal entanglement and once referred to it as "spooky action at a distance." In the words of Jeff Kimble, a professor of physics at Caltech, "Entanglement means if you tickle one the other one laughs."[2] Are the similarities between us and subatomic particles purely metaphorical, or are we living in a holographic reality in which the same principles apply at the interpersonal level? Could there be a parallel experience of two people who have shared a deep affinity and subsequently have instantaneous awareness of each other's experiences across the miles?

INTIMATE CONNECTIONS

The possibility of this was shown in a fascinating experiment conducted by Dr. Jacobo Grinberg-Zylberbaum, a psychology professor at the National Autonomous University of Mexico. In his laboratory, Grinberg-Zylberbaum instructed two young lovers to meditate closely together for twenty minutes. They were then separated into distant, sealed rooms where each was wired to electronic equipment so their brain waves could be monitored. Next, researchers stimulated one of the partners with weak electric shocks to the fingers, flashes of light, and sounds. Amazingly, the brain waves of the other partner in the distant room responded *at the same time*—as though he or she, too, were being stimulated.[3] There are other studies as well showing this phenomenon.

A particularly intriguing view of how such entanglement might occur between partners has been offered recently by the German researcher Harald Walach in his theory of how healers might exert influence across distance. He suggests that under certain circumstances, the human mind by itself may be able to intentionally form a quantum system with another. Intention, ritual, or prayer might be "devices" by which a person can establish entanglement with another wherein together they comprise a single system—at least temporarily. It is in that state of unity that the miracle of healing somehow unfolds.[4]

It's important to note here that we're not talking about one person's transmitting energy to another in the sense of an exchange of bioenergy, chi, or life energy, although this certainly could happen if the two parties were in each other's physical presence. Rather, the point is that as one unified system or "being," there is no "transfer" of energy or intention or anything else because there is nowhere to transfer it from or to—only one "being" is present.

According to Walach's theory, healers' effects in recipients would occur in *correlation* with this state of entanglement. The healing is not actually *caused* by the healer because there is no separation, no time lag, no cause-effect sequence; it is simultaneous. He describes this as "a correlational change in state of one remote part of a system."[5]

Walach is careful to acknowledge several unproven presuppositions on which this idea is based. The first is that it is possible for entanglement to exist between two entities that are much larger than subatomic particles—specifically, two human beings. The second is that boundaries can be formed that are strong enough to hold the two people together as a system on the quantum level and allow entanglement to occur. Perhaps rituals requiring sharply focused attention and intention of the parties involved may be strong enough to achieve this.

The third is that there are "complementary variables"—variables that work together and mutually reinforce each other—within the two-person system that allow for entanglement. As Walach explains, the sequence might look something like this: The healer first creates a boundary encompassing the two people and then performs a form of imagery or ritual that is complementary to the diseased condition of the recipient. This might involve an active kind of imagery such as sucking or drawing the disease process out of the patient and then visualizing the patient healed or blessed with the desired outcome. If this is done with complete faith and belief in the process, it qualifies as "complementary" to the diseased state of the recipient.

Walach observes, "There certainly remains a lot to understand, and it is by no means clear which [criteria] actually fulfill the condition of complementarity. But the nice thing about this model is that there may even be multiple ways of reconstructing complementarity, and not only one single and correct one."[6] His work is based on a healer's intentionally creating a temporary bond with a healee for the purpose of doing the healing work. Our interest, of course, is in how these concepts might apply in your relationship with your partner. It is easy to see how through living together, and especially through meditating or praying together over time, the quality of the bond that Walach is referring to could occur naturally.

CAUSATION OR CORRELATION?

What, then, could we say is the "cause" of distant healing? It seems apparent that an intention on the part of the healer to "entangle" with a recipient and unite with him or her in a single system sets the process in motion. In that sense, you could say that the intentionality of the healer is what precipitates the process. However, once the system has been formed, the healer no longer exists as a separate individual.

What happens within this system, of course, is a mystery. Walach suggests that our beliefs about "causing" healing in another, or about strong intentions, energies, or vibrations, might serve no purpose other than to simply distract our minds—give us something to think about—so that they won't interfere with the deeper process of entanglement. At any rate, he concludes that "it might be necessary for practitioners to think and operate in terms of causality and locality, but crucial for researchers and theoreticians not to be sidetracked by that causalist talk [and] look into the true nature of what lies at the heart of all matter."[7]

A Look at the Evidence

There is, of course, controversy among scientists about whether distant influence is possible and whether it should be regarded as a valid topic of study. The main problem on which critics focus is the lack of an obvious mechanism of action—one that can be broken down, studied, and measured objectively in a laboratory. Without such a mechanism, they argue, any positive findings of studies must be the result of random chance, flawed research methods, or even outright fraud (which, unfortunately, is suspected in isolated cases[8]). Perhaps someday quantum physics will evolve to a point at which it can provide fully satisfying explanations. Or it may well be that distant healing is best regarded as a phenomenon that cannot be fully explained by a scientific paradigm whose tools are, after all, products of and confined to the physical dimension.

Efforts to study distant healing with scientific methods have been burdened by several challenges that make it difficult to come up with a consensus on what science can tell us. One problem is that of the relationship between healer and recipient. Almost all studies use "professional" or "anonymous" healers who work on recipients at a distance, who are unknown to the recipients, and whom the recipients never see or meet. Several studies have used distant anonymous prayer by individuals or by groups to pray for recipients who are strangers to those doing the praying. This works well for having a blinded study—one in which the recipients don't know when or whether they are receiving the intervention. However, if the notion of entanglement is viable, then one can easily see how studies could get differing results depending on the relationship involved. Indeed, to the extent that an intimate loving relationship is essential for entanglement to occur, one might expect negative findings in all studies that use anonymous healers.

Another issue is standardization of techniques. Techniques vary widely across studies, from prayer to visualization to altered states, and are often not clearly described, making it difficult to arrive at a consensus of findings.

Then there is lack of consistency in the qualities of "healers." Some studies use healers who represent a mix of religious, shamanic, and secular schools of energy healing.[9] One used groups of people who merely had espoused a strong personal belief that God is responsive to prayers for healing.[10] None have looked closely at skill levels of healers or personality differences among them.

Finally there is the matter of placebo effects. As you will see later, simply knowing or believing that one is a recipient of another's healing intentions can be beneficial. This may make it difficult to attribute any effects to the healer or the technique used.

"REMOTE INFLUENCE"

For distant healing to occur, there would have to be some possibility of exerting influence on another person over distance—what scientists call "remote influence." Whether such influence might translate into healing is another matter. But several well-controlled studies have shown that influence of one person on another across distance is possible. Much of the early work in this field was done using "healing analog" experiments typically involving biofeedback devices the measuring electrical resistance of the skin, muscle tension, or brain waves) to detect effects in recipients from the efforts of "psychics" or healers attempting to influence them from a distance.

Typically, a recipient would be sitting quietly in a lab, wired to the devices, and a "healer" in a remote location would, at prescribed times unknown to the recipient, use mental intention to attempt to influence the recipient's functioning. This is sometimes referred to as "transpersonal imagery" and is based on the assumption that information can be transmitted from the consciousness of one person to the physical body of another (for example, imaging another person's becoming more relaxed or more stimulated). Over thirty well-designed experiments in this area have demonstrated that such remote influence can alter another's bodily systems.[11]

An illustrative example of this work was conducted by psychologist Jeanne Achterberg, PhD, and her colleagues using functional magnetic resonance imaging (fMRI) to explore the effects of distant intentionality on brain functions in recipients. Eleven local healers from the island of Hawaii who claimed to have distant healing abilities participated. This use of multiple healers was smart because the findings didn't have to hinge on results from just one particular individual, as has often been the case in other studies.

Each healer chose a recipient with whom he or she felt "an intuitive sense of connection" (entanglement, perhaps?) and to whom he or she would direct healing intentions. Each recipient was placed in an fMRI scanner and isolated from all forms of sensory contact with the healer. Then the healer projected distant healing intentions for the recipient at random two-minute intervals. The recipient had no idea when the intentions were being used or not used. The fMRI data from all the healer-recipient pairs were then combined for statistical analysis. Highly significant differences were seen in brain stimulation for the recipients during the periods when healing intention was being used, compared to the periods when it was not. The brain areas showing stimulation included the anterior and middle cingulate area, precuneus, and frontal area.[12]

We don't know exactly how—or whether—the stimulation of these areas might translate into healing outcomes, but the fact that it showed up at all is in itself an affirmation that there is a pathway for interpersonal influence across distance. The study raises interesting questions about the role of relationship: since the healers chose their recipients rather than being assigned someone with whom they felt no familiarity, it may well be that a preexisting sense of connection is a determinant of whether distant effects might occur. It follows that a couple in an intimate relationship may already have these conditions well established.

HEALTH EFFECTS

To show that remote influence is possible is one thing, but to demonstrate healing effects is quite another. Humans are obviously very complex, multisystemic beings, and healing is a very complex multilevel phenomenon. Objective reviews of the state of the science agree that there is insufficient data to prove whether, or when, distant healing can be counted on.[13]

Small studies have shown mixed results. For example, a study with 40 alcoholic patients attending a public substance abuse program looked for impact of distant prayer on drinking behavior six months beyond treatment but did not find positive benefits.[14] Another with 36 children in psychiatric treatment used distant anonymous prayer but found no positive effects.[15] One well-designed study of 120 patients with chronic neuropathic pain used anonymous distant healing intention by trained healers but found no significant impact.[16] A well-designed study examined the effects of distant healing by experienced healers on the size of skin warts (a condition known to respond to hypnotic suggestion) and found no effect.[17]

On the positive side, in a study of fourteen diabetes patients, researchers found that during the assigned intervals of distant healing, subjects' levels of fructosamine (an indicator of blood glucose) were significantly reduced, and after the period of distant healing ended, the levels rose once again.[18] Positive results were also seen in a well-designed study with forty adult psychiatric inpatients being treated for depression: a reduction in symptoms occurred after anonymous distant healing intention.[19] Another study with eight healthy college students found that distant prayer seemed to reduce anxiety over time.[20] A study with eighteen children with leukemia who received daily prayer over fifteen months found a slightly lower death rate.[21] Small studies must always be considered speculative, though, regardless of their findings.

Several large studies have used anonymous distant healing with cardiac disease, but they, too, have had mixed results. For example, two large trials found reductions in complications and in number of days of hospitalization,[22] while another actually found an *increase* in the rate of complications.[23] Other large studies have found no effect.[24] A study with hypertension patients suggested that anonymous distant healing might contribute to reduced blood pressure—specifically, a decrease in systolic blood pressure—but flaws in the design made conclusions unclear.[25]

Two particularly well-designed studies have been done at the California Pacific Medical Center in San Francisco using distant healing intention for HIV/AIDS patients, also with mixed results. One found beneficial impacts on illness severity, need for medical attention, and mood.[26] The second, larger study did not find such benefits. However, it did have one intriguing finding: *those receiving distant healing were significantly more likely to guess that they had been receiving it* than were those in the no-treatment group.[27]

What can we glean from the research? The inconsistency of results does not mean that distant healing cannot or does not work, only that there is a great deal we don't know that needs to be explored. Distant influences are possible, but the conditions under which they might translate into healing are still ambiguous. Factors that could account for inconsistent findings range from how much or how long healing intention was used to the choice of outcome measures, healers' techniques, the relationship between the healer and recipient, training, emotional maturity, and even personality quirks. And if, indeed, we are dealing with a phenomenon that crosses multiple dimensions of reality, there may even be factors on the "other side" we will never understand.

The elephant standing in the room is the studies' use of anonymous healers and *the absence of a personal relationship between healers and recipients*. This does not reflect real life. It attempts to separate out the phenomenon of healing intention from the context of relationship in which it naturally occurs, where it is truly genuine and grounded in a history between two people. In real life, loved ones who are entangled with one another pray for one another or hold healing intentions for one another, and do so frequently—maybe even continuously—over time, resulting in a far greater "dose" than anything that has ever been studied in any of the research. The evidence shows that there are pathways for influence but tells us nothing about the value of distant healing intention between people in a relationship.

Seen in that light, your use of distant healing practices may be better regarded as faith-based than science-based—or a combination of the two. Certainly the few positive studies, and especially the laboratory studies documenting the reality of distant connectedness, should reinforce a sense of hope and possibility in anyone who wants to have an impact on a loved one at a distance. The integrative, "cocreative" perspective would remind you that you do not control the results, and certainly you should not feel a sense of failure if you don't get the results you want in a given situation.

Personal Rewards

An often-overlooked aspect of distant healing is that while your efforts might bring benefits to your partner, you will also be benefiting yourself. As we've already seen, a common source of distress in care partners is a sense of powerlessness and despair over a perceived inability to influence the patient's condition, reduce his or her suffering, or contribute to the healing process. Psychologists refer to this as low "self-efficacy" in the support role, meaning that you lack self-confidence or belief in your ability to make a difference. By practicing distant healing for your partner, you know you are doing something that may make a difference.

Another way you benefit is the relaxation and comfort you can gain from the techniques themselves. Many studies have shown that meditative and prayerful practices help generate relaxation, calm, and peace in the practitioner.[28]

Beyond those relatively general benefits, there is now even more evidence that focusing specifically on the well-being of another can have added effects. Father Seán ÓLaoire, who is both a Catholic priest and a clinical psychologist in Palo Alto, California, conducted a randomized controlled trial of the effects of intercessory prayer for others on self-esteem, anxiety, and depression. In a one-hour workshop, volunteers were trained in a simple technique of prayerful intention for others. Over the next twelve weeks, they prayed fifteen minutes daily for anonymous recipients known to them only by a photo and first name. At follow-up, those who prayed for others had significant improvements in their own levels of self-esteem, anxiety, and depression.[29] Perhaps it is the inner state of relaxation and peace the practice evoked that is the source of benefit; or the experience of compassionate, selfless action; or perhaps there is a further explanation in terms of the dynamics of entanglement yet to be charted. Regardless, it's a win-win situation for you and your partner.

The Essential Tools

While we may never fully understand the mystery of distant healing, we can learn from people who seem to be adept at it. What are the qualities that reputed healers have in common? There is no reason to believe these qualities would not be available to all of us.

Marilyn Schlitz, PhD, of the Institute of Noetic Sciences, and the late Elisabeth Targ, MD, of California Pacific Medical Center in San Francisco, undertook the challenge of identifying the common elements of successful healers and, in NIH-sponsored research, training laypeople in these skills. As part of their background exploration, they studied the curricula of a variety of healing traditions and training programs that teach distant healing. They found what they concluded to be the common premise underlying distant healing across all traditions that use it, regardless of the form: *compassionate intention*. They further identified three common elements that seem to underlie the preparation of healers to practice with compassionate intention. These are (1) the cultivation of attention, (2) the development of compassion, and (3) belief or confidence in the method.[30] These are qualities that any of us can develop.

ATTENTION

"Attention" involves your being in a state of concentration and nondistractibility. What we're really striving for is what could be called "sustained attention." This is commonly taught as the first step before many approaches to healing and may involve a period of relaxation or "centering" to enhance concentration on the process.[31]

Attention is a quality of mind that you can easily cultivate by practicing meditation or other ways of focusing your mind without wavering. For example, attention is the basis of mindfulness meditation, which involves focusing on your breath, a sound, a chant or phrase, or some other object of focus. In essence, "mindfulness" means that your mind is full of attention on what you have chosen as your focus.

For any form of distant healing, it is a good idea to prepare yourself by spending five to ten minutes just centering yourself. Here are instructions for a simple centering process:

1. Sit in an upright posture with your eyes closed and rest your hands in your lap, open with palms facing upward. Imagine a string connecting the center of the earth to a star high up in the heavens, and passing straight up through the center of your body and out through the top of your head. Move your body slightly from side to side and front to back around this string until you find that point of perfect balance.

2. Now take a couple of long, full, complete breaths and exhale fully. Let your breath become the center of your attention. Notice your body's subtle movements with each breath; notice the texture or temperature of the air, or other nuances of the breath as it moves in and out. Focus all your attention on the experience of each breath as fully as you can.

3. Whenever thoughts arise, do not engage them but gently return your attention back to your breath. There's no need to try to stop your mind or fight it. Thoughts will come and go, so the point is that when they do arise, you simply let them pass by like birds across the sky while you return your attention to the experience of each breath.

This practice will enable you to become calm, centered, and more present for the distant healing efforts you wish to explore.

COMPASSIONATE OR EMPATHIC RESPONSE

The second element that seems to underlie the preparation of healers to practice with compassionate intention refers to your experience of selfless love and care for the other's suffering.[32] Various traditions teach practices to increase your sense of love and care for the other, to experience "self" as extending beyond your skin, and to have a sense of connection with the other.[33] Compassion is also related to empathy—the ability to feel what the other is feeling, suggesting a dissolution of boundaries between yourself and your partner.[34]

You can strengthen your ability to feel compassion by first setting your intention to do so and then being in situations that stimulate a sense of empathy and compassion. You may not need to look beyond your relationships with your partner, your family, friends, or neighbors to find opportunities to cultivate compassion within yourself. Or many forms of volunteer work in your own community can help you develop this.

BELIEF OR CONFIDENCE IN THE METHOD

Finally, in order for your efforts to be effective, you must believe or have confidence in the method you are using. Strong faith and belief in the technique will help you invest your full attention in the process and assuage self-doubts that might dilute your efforts. In their own training program, Schlitz and Targ, who were themselves leading-edge researchers in this area, actually incorporated a review of research findings on distant healing for participants.

The message I hope you will take from part 5 is that you probably already have the prerequisites in place to positively benefit your partner by using distant healing practices. The sense of connection between you, open communication about your efforts, and the compassionate intention that exists within you for your partner are enough to find satisfaction and reward in using any of the methods that follow.

28

Transforming Suffering

THE THOUGHT OF SOMEHOW TAKING YOUR PARTNER'S SUF-
fering upon yourself might seem at first overwhelming. And, yet, many
traditions share a common understanding that the human heart is a
transformative organ—like a crucible that can transform energy from
negative to positive, from darkness to light, or in the metaphor of the
ancient alchemists, from base metals into gold.

There is a very direct and particularly empowering meditation on
transforming another's suffering called *tonglen,* a traditional Tibetan
Buddhist practice to cultivate and strengthen the heart's ability to feel
compassion for the suffering of others. The practice involves the simple
use of intention and the breath. Traditionally, it is taught with a focus on
the suffering of all beings, but it can be focused on individuals as well.

Begin with a period of meditation to calm and center yourself, perhaps using loving-kindness meditation. Then, on the in-breath, imagine
you are breathing the suffering of your partner into your heart, where it
is transformed. On the out-breath, imagine you are pouring out peace
and healing (tonglen literally means "giving and receiving" in the Tibetan
language) directed back toward your partner, and imagine that he or she
is breathing it in.

In *The Tibetan Book of Living and Dying,* the contemporary Buddhist scholar and teacher Sogyal Rinpoche describes this practice in rich
detail. He observes:

> In the Tonglen practice of giving and receiving, we *take* on, *through*
> *compassion,* all the various mental and physical sufferings of all
> beings: their fear, frustration, pain, anger, guilt, bitterness, doubt,
> and rage, and we *give* them, *through love,* all our happiness, well
> being, peace of mind, healing, and fulfillment.[1]

He recounts the story of an eleventh-century master named Geshe
Chechawa who taught this revered practice to lepers as a path to their

own enlightenment. The testimony to the transformative power of the practice was that with time, as a by-product, some were cured of their disease. Sogyal Rinpoche also writes of people with AIDS using this practice and seeing their own suffering transformed.

Remember that you are not absorbing or retaining your partner's suffering permanently within yourself. Rather, you envision transforming it into love and light, which you send back with your out-breath. This is a wonderful way to increase your confidence in your own heart and strengthen your capacity for compassion—for yourself, for others, and for the world.

For more information on tonglen practice, see *Always Maintain a Joyful Mind,* by Pema Chödrön, which includes an audio CD of guided instruction in tonglen practice.

29

Transpersonal Imagery

RELAXATION AND PEACE

TRANSPERSONAL IMAGERY IS SIMPLY A PROCESS OF IMAGINING what you would like your partner to be experiencing, and focusing your attention on projecting these intentions while in a meditative state. It is based on the principle that you and your partner are a quantum system in which strongly held intentionality in one part of the system can influence the other part.

You can use transpersonal imagery in much the same way people use imagery and visualization to promote self-healing—in fact, it is best to communicate with your partner about what specific images he or she prefers to use and would like you to reinforce. This way there is concurrence between the two of you, and your partner will appreciate this sense of reinforcement.

The most basic kind of healing imagery is that pertaining to relaxation and peace. Hundreds of studies have documented the health benefits of the relaxation response. It is not only an antidote to stress but also has tangible physiological benefits for many bodily systems, including the immune, nervous, and cardiovascular systems. It is a fundamental tool for coping with emotional challenges of illness, and it can also encourage the body's healing responses.

Relaxation is something you can easily visualize for your partner in a variety of ways. Here are two examples.

Light Golden Mist

Begin by closing your eyes and taking a few long, slow, relaxing breaths. Take time to put yourself into a state of relaxation and peace using whatever methods work best for you.

Now imagine your partner surrounded by a light golden mist. Imagine that this light golden mist dissolves away any tension, anxiety, distress, or discomfort in your partner and brings a state of deep relaxation and peace.

Imagine that each breath your partner takes draws in the light golden mist and sends it throughout his or her circulatory system, bringing a deep sense of relaxation and letting go of all tension throughout the body. The light golden mist is reaching into every cell, and every cell becomes deeply calm and relaxed. Imagine that with this state of deep relaxation, all your partner's healing mechanisms are able to work at their maximum.

Relaxation Breath

Use your own breath to bring a state of deep relaxation and peace within yourself. Putting all your attention on each breath, imagine that there is a hollow pipe extending up and down through the center of your body, from your pelvis up to your throat. Using a series of long, slow, satisfying breaths, breathe in a way that feels comforting and gratifying. Breathe each breath up and down through the length of this pipe, and each time you notice that your attention has wandered, simply bring your attention back to the breath.

Let each breath be long, slow, and deep. You might imagine each in-breath and each out-breath as having three segments (beginning, middle, end) and just mentally note each segment, as each in-breath and each out-breath passes through you.

After breathing this way for a while, when you feel you have attained a state of relaxation and peace within yourself, imagine you are now breathing this same breath for your partner. This deliberate, comforting, and satisfying breath is moving through your partner's body this same way, bringing the same sense of relaxation and peace you are feeling.

30

Transpersonal Imagery

HEALING PROCESSES

FOR IMAGERY FOCUSED ON SPECIFIC HEALING PROCESSES, the place to begin is talking with your partner about what kind of images he or she would like you to use. As I will explain in chapter 35, your partner's simply knowing he or she is the object of your distant healing efforts can in itself be a powerful source of support and comfort. The knowledge that you are using images compatible with how your partner wants to think of these processes in his or her own body will only add confidence for both of you and is certainly preferable to unilaterally coming up with your own images that may not resonate with your partner.

People differ in their preferences as to how literal or symbolic they like their healing imagery to be. There is no reason to believe one is superior to the other. What matters is to use imagery that helps to generate a feeling of confidence and positive expectancy. It is these qualities that seem to be the common threads in studies that show imagery to be an effective healing intervention. You and your partner can formulate imagery for any healing process desired. As with all other forms of distant healing, for each of these, always begin with a period of centering and preparation within yourself. Here are a few examples.

Wound Healing

Picture your partner's wound or incision in front of you and imagine what healing processes are going on in the background. You might imagine the macrophages of the immune system (the white cells that devour unhealthy material) clearing away any debris, infection, or dead tissue so that clean, pink, healthy tissue can take its place. Picture the macrophages devouring anything that needs to be removed and carrying it away.

Imagine fresh, young, pink, healthy tissue filling in the wound and taking the proper shape and consistency so that area of your partner's body returns to its natural healthy state.

If there is an incision or a break in the skin, imagine it closing and the skin knitting back together again to form a smooth and resilient closure on the area. Then imagine any scar tissue slowly dissolving until it disappears.

Immune Stimulation

If your partner has a condition that requires greater immune activity, such as cancer or infection, talk together about what symbolic imagery he or she might like you to use for this. For example, you could imagine the white cells massing in areas of cancer or infection like piranha or wolves and devouring any unwanted material, leaving behind only clean, fresh, healthy tissue. (See "Tumors" on page 140 for alternatives.)

Immune Modulation

Some illnesses are a result of aberrant responses of the immune system and would not call for imagery of heightened activity. In these cases, you and your partner can use imagery of the immune system's coming back into proper harmony and balance rather than being stimulated to higher activity. For example, chronic fatigue syndrome involves an unregulated release of cytokines (hormones produced by the immune system) that cause the symptoms of fatigue. Autoimmune illnesses like multiple sclerosis or rheumatoid arthritis involve the immune system's attacking the body's own healthy tissues.

You can practice imagery of the immune system's becoming more relaxed, calm, and peaceful. As you take long, slow, relaxing breaths, imagine you are breathing this same relaxation into your partner's immune system. Imagine that the white cells are breathing along with you and that the white cells themselves are becoming calmer, more peaceful, and more relaxed with each breath. Know that with this calm and relaxation comes clearer vision and greater discernment, so that your partner's white cells more clearly see where they are truly needed and retreat from places where they are not needed.

Allergies and asthma are also conditions with a component of overactive immune responses. Here is another situation in which imagery of the immune system's becoming calmer and more relaxed may be preferred.

Tumors

Imagery for reducing or eliminating tumors can be done in a variety of ways. One is to imagine heightened immune activity around the tumor, as described above, with white cells massing around it and clearing it away in a methodical, piecemeal, and deliberate manner.

Some people, however, do not like the use of combative or warlike imagery in reference to their body. Your partner might prefer that you imagine the tumor melting like butter or ice, or slowly dissolving. Or you could imagine your partner's body being filled with a golden healing light, like the sun, that is overwhelming any areas of darkness, melting them or drying them out, and shrinking them down to nothing with the help of its warmth or vibrant light.

Cardiovascular Conditions

If your partner has heart disease or hypertension, any imagery related to relaxation and peace would be relevant. Your partner's circulatory system is lined with thousands of miles of smooth muscular tissue that can contract or relax depending on states of stress or relaxation. Anytime during your day, you can take time to go into a relaxing meditation yourself as preparation and then imagine a feeling of relaxation and peace spreading throughout your partner's entire cardiovascular system, encouraging smooth, even, and relaxed heart function.

Imagine the walls of your partner's arteries becoming flexible and slippery, any unwanted deposits dissolving away. Imagine his or her blood pressure relaxing and turning downward toward normal.

Chronic Pain

If your partner has a chronic pain condition, this is another case in which supporting generalized relaxation and peace can help. This is because tension or stress exacerbates pain levels, while relaxation reduces them.

Often a person in chronic pain develops muscular holding patterns to immobilize the affected area and defend against the pain, but this can actually make it worse by reducing circulation of blood and lymph to and through the area.

Here you can rely on the general imagery for encouraging relaxation and peace throughout your partner's body, and you can also visualize healing energy, light, or nutrients flowing through the painful area to promote healing.

Some chronic pain conditions involve aberrant responses of the nervous system and are not caused by local tissue damage. For example, fibromyalgia pain is felt bodywide, but the pain sensations mainly result from a malfunction in processing sensation—usually as a result of some shock or trauma to the nervous system (such as an automobile accident). In this case, what is needed is healing of the nervous system itself. In addition to the generalized benefits of imagery for relaxation and peace, you could also visualize the vast network of the nervous system in your partner's body and imagine directing your breath throughout that network. Imagine that your breath is bringing calm, peace, and relaxation throughout your partner's nervous system and that this is helping it restore harmony, balance, and healthy functioning.

Alternatively, you could imagine your partner's nervous system being filled with a golden healing light. Each breath you take is reinforcing the integrity and strength of that golden healing light as it heals your partner's nervous system all the way from the brain to the tips of the fingers and toes.

31

Transpersonal Imagery

SUCCESSFUL SURGERY

Surgery can be stressful for the care partner as well as the recipient, but the good news is that it is a single event that you can prepare for in advance. There are many studies documenting the effectiveness of using imagery and relaxation exercises to prepare for surgery. Patients have been able to influence their level of complications and blood loss and the speed of their recovery.

You can discuss together a vision of how you both would like the surgery to proceed, from preparation to recovery, so that you are each holding and reinforcing the same imagery during this time. Here is another time when it may be particularly supportive to your partner to know about your distant healing efforts. You reinforce your partner's own efforts to prepare, and your intentions from a distance may further contribute to the outcomes you both desire. Here are a few ideas you can develop together.

Preparation of the Surgical Team

Visualize the members of the surgical team all surrounded and filled by light. Imagine that they all have clear vision, skillful hands, and are guided by your highest good in every way. Imagine that they are all filled with peace as they work with your partner's body.

Cooperation of the Body

Visualize your partner's entire body relaxed, peaceful, and welcoming to the work of the surgery. Imagine the body cooperating in every way, including with minimal loss of blood—imagine the surgeon being amazed at how little blood is lost and how little need there is for transfusion, maybe even none at all.

Gratitude to the Body

If a part of your partner's body is being removed during surgery, express gratitude for its service in the past and thank the body for releasing this now unneeded part easily and gracefully. Imagine your partner's body willingly relinquishing the old material.

Recovery

Imagine your partner awakening from the surgery feeling confident and very much alive and well. See the two of you along with the surgeon marveling at how well the surgery went and how little discomfort your partner is feeling.

Imagine your partner's body easily knitting back together at the surgical site. The surgical wound is healing rapidly, and integrity is quickly restored to that area of the body. Imagine fresh supplies of life energy and nutrients circulating easily through the area, reinforcing its healing and integrity.

32

Transpersonal Imagery

EFFECTIVE TREATMENT

IF YOUR PARTNER IS RECEIVING A FORM OF MEDICAL TREAT-
ment, you can join him or her in visualizing it working in the optimal
way. This may be particularly supportive in treatments that are arduous
or have side effects, such as chemotherapy and radiation, which are discussed below. You should discuss together what kinds of imagery would
help your partner feel confidence in the treatment and maintain a positive attitude toward it, as positive expectancy is known to influence the
effectiveness of medical treatment.

Chemotherapy

Cancer chemotherapy is often accompanied by unpleasant side effects
that make it a challenge to maintain a positive attitude toward receiving
it. You and your partner can work out imagery to help maintain a positive
receptivity and acceptance toward it, knowing that in the long run, it will
be of benefit and worth the short-term side effects.

For example, imagine the chemotherapy as a cleansing potion that is
dissolving and removing unwanted material from the body, all of which
is released through natural elimination. Imagine that your partner's organs of detoxification, the liver and kidneys, are filtering out any wastes
from the work of the chemotherapy and the drug itself when its work
is done. And imagine that your partner's tissues are recovering quickly
from any temporary adverse effects, repairing any damage, rebuilding,
and regaining vibrant health—in between rounds of chemotherapy as
well as after it has been completed.

Most side effects of chemotherapy are reduced by relaxation because
it helps your partner to be in a less reactive state. You can use the gener-

alized relaxation imagery to support this state in your partner when you are apart.

Radiation Therapy

Radiation is another treatment with some unpleasant side effects, though they tend to be more short-lived. Essentially, radiation therapy works by killing cancer cells; collateral damage is done to healthy tissues in the area, but these healthy tissues heal and grow back after the treatment.

Side effects of radiation therapy vary widely and can include pain, burning, or digestive disturbances, depending on the area of the body being treated. In all cases, a common side effect is generalized fatigue. Here is another instance in which imagery to encourage relaxation and peace can be supportive for your partner, as relaxation will help reduce the severity of discomfort and will also help to speed healing in the areas of collateral damage to healthy tissues. As for fatigue, you might take a few minutes in your day to visualize your partner breathing in fully, getting the maximum benefit from each breath, so that vital energy in the body can be replenished.

Other Treatments

You and your partner, as a quantum system, can come up with imagery for just about any other form of medical treatment. Discuss what your partner wants the treatment to accomplish and what he or she would like you to visualize when you are apart. Remember that imagery can be based on literal understanding of desired treatment effects, or symbolic images that represent effective action of the treatment in your partner's body.

33

Prayer

PRAYER HAS A SPECIAL PLACE IN THE WORLD OF DISTANT healing. It differs from other forms of distant healing in that it does not presume that you are exerting healing influence directly on your partner. Instead, it involves asking for a higher power to intercede (the root of "intercessory") on your behalf. The existence of an all-powerful force beyond us is, of course, the basis of a religious perspective on life, and the world's religions universally celebrate the healing power of the Absolute in whatever form they conceive it.

Implicit in the experience of prayer is an element of surrender. You are not exerting influence through a hypothetical quantum system in which you and your partner are one. Rather, you are acknowledging a higher power as the source of intervention. And you can't know what the will of that higher power is or what it may have in "mind" for you or your partner. From that perspective, you can't truly know what is in your partner's highest good. You can't know the details of the larger plan for you, your partner, or the world.

Depending on your personal beliefs, or perhaps at different times in your partner's healing journey, you may feel more drawn to prayer than to some of the other forms of distant healing. For example, acute crises or times when dying is a possibility naturally evoke a greater openness to seeking communion with a higher power.

Some care partners feel more confident with a daily practice that combines multiple forms of distant healing support for their loved one. Lydia, whose husband, Ralph, is recovering from quadruple-bypass surgery, describes her own practice this way: "Each morning I begin with a prayer of gratitude for the day. I follow this with loving-kindness meditation for about twenty minutes. Then I pray for my own health and Ralph's continued healing, and I always end with 'Thy will be done.'"

Lydia's approach illustrates an important point about prayer. In his abundant writings on the research dealing with prayer, physician and visionary Larry Dossey has helped to make an important distinction between directive and nondirective prayer. Directive prayers are those in which we ask for a specific desired outcome, such as "Make her cancer go away," "Help him pull through this surgery," or "Make the clot shrink and disappear."

Behind such requests is a presumption that the Absolute can and might grant us what we desire because we are sincerely asking for it—that our very asking incurs some favor that just might yield the response we want.

Nondirective prayer is in a sense more mature and humble. It does not presume that we can know what is best or right. As Lydia showed, we can certainly ask for what we want, but at the same time, we recognize there is a much larger picture than what we can grasp. Nondirective prayer is best characterized by the intentions of "If it be Thy will," "Thy will be done," and "May the highest good prevail."

The element of surrender to higher wisdom and higher power can be a relief, in that you don't have to figure out what exactly is the right thing to pray for. You don't have to have a sophisticated understanding of your partner's medical condition, and you can't do it wrong. In contrast with other forms of distant healing, nondirective prayer is more restful: you can relax in the knowledge that you are aligning yourself with the will of the Absolute. In trusting that there is a higher intelligence working behind the scenes, you are off the hook.

PART SIX

Affirmative Communication

34

Well-Chosen Words

COMMUNICATION, THE ESSENCE OF RELATIONSHIP, TAKES ON new dynamics and new importance when illness enters the picture. The stresses of illness—however subtle—can influence the climate of a relationship and color its communication over time. Communication can be good medicine, or it can be an added stressor that makes things worse for both partners. Many couples facing illness together wonder, "What are our needs for communication?" "What kind of communication is most helpful and supportive?" and "How can our communication benefit us both?"

Much of what we know about communication in illness has been learned from couples living with cancer. This is because of its prevalence and the fact that cancer research is so well funded in comparison to many other conditions, giving behavioral scientists more opportunity to use it as a model to probe the psychological aspects of living with illness. Nevertheless, the insights gained apply to couples dealing with illness of all kinds, since the core communication issues that arise transcend any specific diagnosis. In part 6, I'd like to review some key insights from research into couple communication in the context of illness and then look at strategies you can use to make communication a real tool of support for your partner.

As you'll see in the discussion of studies below, supportive communication sets in motion a chain of influences that will ultimately contribute to improved well-being for your partner. Whenever the effects of communication and relationship quality on illness are explored, the same set of linkages comes up, regardless of what the specific illness might be. The linkages look something like this:

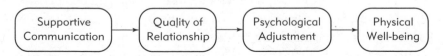

There's a welcome bonus in all this for you as the care partner. Your efforts to practice supportive communication will only strengthen the quality of your relationship, which, in turn, will reinforce your own psychological well-being and quite possibly your own health.

A Look at the Evidence

WHAT IS SUPPORTIVE?

Some pretty clear guidelines have come to light in recent years as to what kind of communication people with illness find most helpful and supportive from their mate. Some of the best work in this area was done at Fox Chase Cancer Center in Philadelphia by Sharon Manne and her colleagues. In one study, they interviewed 148 couples on videotape as they had two different kinds of conversations—one discussing illness-related issues and another discussing a general, more neutral topic. The patients also completed questionnaires to measure their level of psychological distress and their satisfaction with the relationship after each conversation. The videos were later analyzed to understand how the partners were responding as the patients disclosed their thoughts and feelings.

During the illness-related discussions (the more stressful topic), the patients had less distress if their partners responded in three ways. First was "reciprocal self-disclosure"—that is, the partner's sharing his or her own feelings and concerns—in effect, matching the level of sharing of feelings being done by the patient. Second was responding with humor—not minimizing the situation but using humor as a sort of escape valve to relieve tension. And third was the partner's willingness to be present with the patient and with the mutual expression of feelings instead of just jumping ahead into looking for solutions. When discussing the neutral topic, which didn't have the emotional charge of the stressful topic, the patients weren't affected nearly as much by how the partner responded.[1]

This study tells us that patients are helped most by partners who are good listeners, express their own feelings, use humor, and don't charge ahead into problem-solving mode. These responses help reduce psychological distress, which makes it harder to adjust to illness.

Two other studies illustrate variations on the theme of partner self-disclosure. In one study of 98 women with breast cancer, patients reported feeling their relationship had more intimacy the more their partners disclosed their own feelings. The women said they felt more accepted, understood, and cared for with such disclosure.[2] In the other study, with 113 women with breast cancer, patients described their partners as "good communicators" if they were able to empathize and not withdraw from talking about the emotional aspects and stresses of illness. Patients who were most satisfied with the support they were receiving from their partners were found to have better psychological well-being.[3]

Beyond the willingness to disclose your feelings, researchers at the University of Texas looked at the value of "relationship talk"—keeping a dialogue open about how your relationship is going. In this study, 182 couples participated, half in which one partner had a chronic illness and half in which both partners were well. All couples completed a questionnaire about communication and marital quality. For the couples in which one partner was ill, relationship talk had a greater impact on their ratings of the quality of their relationship than it did for couples in which both partners were healthy.[4]

How often you talk together about the stresses of illness matters, too. This was shown in a study of the effects of the frequency of a couple's communication about illness on depressive feelings. About a month after surgery, 120 breast cancer patients were interviewed to determine frequency of general communication with their partner, frequency of communication specifically about illness, and the women's satisfaction with communication. The results indicated that less communication was associated with higher levels of depression, whereas frequent dialogue about the illness was associated with less depression.[5] And a smaller study of 58 breast illness couples found that in couples who talked more frequently about the illness, *both* the patient and the partner showed better adjustment.[6]

HOW DISCLOSURE HELPS

How can disclosing your feelings and concerns to your mate have such a powerful impact? It seems to have a bonding effect, making couples feel more connected. This was suggested in a study at Duke University Medical Center by Laura Porter and her colleagues, who looked at the connection between disclosure of illness-related concerns and the couple's perception of the quality of their relationship. Forty-seven cancer couples participated in the study. They found that higher disclosure and lower withholding of feelings and concerns were associated with lower psychological distress in both the patient and the partner and higher ratings of relationship quality by both the patient and the partner.[7]

This was confirmed in another study of ninety-five couples living with chronic pain. The patients who were able to talk more frequently about their pain to their partner rated their marital satisfaction higher than patients who talked about their pain less.[8]

Further evidence of a bonding effect comes from a Canadian study of 282 couples with newly diagnosed breast cancer. Forty-two percent of the couples said the illness brought them closer, while in only 6 percent did one partner or the other report feeling distanced, and in less than 1 percent did both partners report feeling distanced. The couples who felt most strongly that they had been brought closer were the ones in which the care partner (1) treated the patient as a confidant, (2) asked her for advice about coping, (3) accompanied her to surgery, and (4) demonstrated increased affection.[9]

Disclosure of emotions also contributes to "posttraumatic growth"—a positive sense of personal learning or development as a result of going through a crisis. This was the conclusion of a study with 162 breast cancer couples a year and a half after initial treatment. Increased emotional sharing was found to contribute to posttraumatic growth in both the patient and the partner.[10]

Needless to say, it is not just female patients who do better when their marital quality is better. For example, a study of 198 male survivors of coronary heart disease found that those men whose relationship quality was higher tended to adjust better psychologically to their illness.[11]

What happens when you withhold your feelings? As you might imagine, this has the opposite effect. A small Swedish study illustrates what can happen when couples are resigned to keeping their feelings to themselves. Researchers looked at communication in nine couples in which the woman had suffered a heart attack and the man was the care partner. In this small group, they observed that each partner wanted to protect the other from becoming emotionally upset. Each thought he or she could sense how the other felt, but at the same time, there was a lack of direct verbal communication about the crisis they had been through together.

In private interviews, the women acknowledged suffering feelings of guilt and shame about being "weak" and "useless" and withholding their feelings from their husbands.[12] This is exactly the kind of avoidance and withholding that can lead each partner to feeling lonely and isolated within the relationship.

A similar kind of resignation was expressed in a group of eighteen women living with men who had sustained severe head injuries. While the women retained a sense of commitment to the relationship into the future, they were particularly distressed with the men's lack of communication about their feelings and rated their marital satisfaction as lower following the injury.[13]

It's not uncommon for one partner to hold off on deciding whether to express feelings depending on what the other does. This was seen in a study of 219 couples with early-stage breast cancer: some of the women waited to see whether they felt their partners were going to be supportive before they decided to express their own feelings.[14]

THREE PATTERNS OF COUPLE COMMUNICATION

Rather than looking simply at the actions of individual partners in a relationship, another way to look at couple communication is to consider patterns, like "protocols," that both people seem to agree to. In a study of 147 breast cancer couples, researchers at Fox Chase Cancer Center looked at each couple as a system to see what kind of overall communication patterns they seemed to follow for dealing with the stresses of illness and its treatments. Both the patients and their partners completed questionnaires while the women were being treated and again nine months later. Questions dealt with communication patterns, distress, and relationship satisfaction.

Three prevailing types of patterns emerged. The first and most successful was called "mutual constructive communication," in which both parties disclosed their feelings and talked openly about the issues facing them together. For couples in which this was the predominant pattern, both the patient and the partner had lower distress and higher relationship satisfaction. These outcomes were even stronger for the patients who were more severely ill.

The second pattern was called "demand-withdraw communication," in which one of the parties would make demands and the other would withdraw in response. In couples who primarily followed this pattern, both the patient and the partner had higher distress and lower relationship satisfaction.

The third pattern seen was "mutual avoidance," in which neither partner would directly engage the issues or their feelings with the other. In couples using this approach, both the patient and the partner had higher distress, but this strategy didn't seem to affect relationship satisfaction either way.[15]

In summary, it's clear that supportive communication can be very good medicine, both for a partner who is ill and for yourself. The basic guidelines can be boiled down to these seven:

1. Listen well.
2. Express your own feelings—treat your partner as a confidant.
3. Use humor when you can.
4. Don't skip over feelings into problem-solving mode.
5. Don't avoid talking about the emotional aspects and stresses of illness.
6. Talk about how your relationship is going ("relationship talk").
7. Talk about the illness as frequently as your partner would like.

Reinforcing a Climate of Healing

The above guidelines speak mostly to the "how" of supportive communication, but there's another dimension that can enrich the "what" that you communicate during the course of everyday life. It involves the flow of positive and affirmative comments between you.

While it is necessary at times in every relationship to address problems and give criticism or advice or to correct your partner, effective communication is primarily positive. Why? One theory is that positive communication creates significantly more "connectivity" between people—that is, it encourages further communication, interaction, and positive emotions—whereas negative communications encourage distancing and erosion of intimacy.[16]

Through observing couples over many years, John Gottman and his colleagues at the University of Washington have found that people's happiness with their relationship can be gauged to a large extent by the *ratio* of positive to negative content in their communications with each other—what researchers now call the Gottman ratio.[17] Specifically, if the ratio is approximately five or more positive statements to each negative statement, couples are more likely to be satisfied with their relationship.

This surplus of positives is important because a single negative comment actually has more enduring impact than a single positive comment: *negative is actually stronger than positive* when it comes to the long-term reverberations of what we communicate. Couples in which the ratio is equal or has more negative than positive comments are likely to be very dissatisfied. Gottman has offered this insight as something couples can use to consciously improve their relationship satisfaction.

This principle was discovered in observing normal couples over time, but as you can imagine, to the extent that illness in a partner contributes to ongoing stress in the background, it might be harder for a couple to keep the ratio well up in positive territory. For this reason, it may be a good idea for you and your partner to be more consciously aware of keeping a flow of positive communication going and in stressful times make extra effort to verbally encourage and compliment each other. If you must criticize or correct your partner, you need to have many positive interactions to make up for that. Giving compliments and praise; expressing appreciation, gratitude, and affection; helping with tasks; and having interesting conversations are all ways to keep the ratio higher up in the positive zone.

This has been a strategy that Kate and Bruce have used spontaneously for years. Kate is suffering from fibromyalgia, a particularly stress-sensitive condition that is seriously aggravated by Bruce's critical and volatile personality. A Vietnam veteran, he has a history of posttraumatic stress disorder (PTSD) and struggles with his own inner turmoil, which frequently comes out as heartless criticism of Kate and hostile teasing directed toward her. What keeps their relationship afloat, as she tells it, is that every day Bruce delivers an abundance of very positive messages. "He's always telling me that he loves me, he thinks I'm cute, thinks I'm adorable, the most beautiful woman in the world, and that he could never live without me." She knows these feelings are genuine, and she feels the same level of devotion toward him. But while she has been making great strides in confronting him and not tolerating his outbursts, she recognizes that progress for him is likely to continue to be slow. The surplus of positive communication is serving them well.

These are good things to practice and should be staples in any relationship. And, in the face of illness, there are some more specific ways you can use such affirmative communication to even greater advantage. In the chapters that follow, I will discuss three simple but powerful ways to expand this form of support for your partner.

35

Sharing Heart's Intentions

IF YOU ARE USING DISTANT HEALING TO SUPPORT YOUR PART-
ner, whether it is Metta, tonglen, prayer, or transpersonal imagery, one
way you can help assure positive results is to simply tell him or her what
you are doing in this regard—or better yet, discuss it together. The reason is simple: knowing that one is the object of another's healing intentions is in itself a powerful influence.

This was the finding of Harald Wiesendanger and his colleagues at the
University of Freiburg in Germany, who studied the effects on recipients
of *knowing* that they were the object of others' efforts to send healing
intentions rather than *not* knowing, as in other studies.[1] In this study, 119
patients with chronic illnesses that had not responded to conventional
treatment (such as migraines, arthritis, or neurological conditions) were
randomly assigned to either be on a waiting list and receive no distant
healing or receive one of three methods of distant healing.

Those in the healing group were divided into three subgroups. In the
first, thirty patients didn't know who was treating them or when, but they
were treated from a distance by three or four different anonymous healers. The second group contained ten patients who were given an amulet
by one healer who invested it with "healing energy," to wear at night. The
third group were twenty patients, each of whom was treated by a healer
with whom they had telephone or in-person contact, though the main
healing activity took place over distance.

The outcome being measured was the patients' quality of life as determined by a scale that rated overall physical, mental, and social functioning. Overall quality of life remained steady in the untreated group but
improved significantly in the patients who were assigned to *any* of the
three protocols of distant healing; there were no differences in effectiveness among the three forms.

This study didn't separate out how much of the improvement might
have been due to the distant healing itself versus the mere power of

suggestion (the placebo effect). But this is not a problem because, in real life, people usually have no reason to hide from each other the fact that they are supporting each other in this way. It affirms the value of the expressions of support that people naturally give each other in times of trauma or illness. To tell your partner "I'll be praying for you" in effect gives him or her two interventions in one. The sense of positive expectancy it inspires in the partner, perhaps even at a subconscious level, may by itself alter his or her emotional well-being, stress level, and perhaps even biochemistry. Add to this any possible effects of the actual prayer itself and you are giving your partner a very healthy dose of support.

36

Coaffirmations

ONE OF THE MOST HELPFUL TOOLS OF MIND-BODY MEDICINE
is the use of affirmations. An affirmation is simply a repeated statement
that expresses an intention regarding something a person wants to have
manifested in his or her life. It may be a change in one's state of health,
a change of behavior, a change of attitude, or some form of outward
success. For example, an affirmation for general well-being might be
"Every day, in every way, I am becoming more and more healthy." For
a successful surgery, one might be "My surgery is going smoothly and
easily, my body is relaxed and peaceful, and my recovery is complete in
every way." These are repeated ten times at one sitting daily, in order
for the intentions to be strengthened and penetrate deeply into your
unconscious mind.

Affirmations work as a form of autosuggestion or self-hypnosis. That
is, by repeating the statement often and over time, the person is, in effect, programming his or her unconscious to adapt to a certain reality.
And, of course, the unconscious mind can influence every cell of the
body through the pathways of the nervous system and the chemical factory of the brain.

To the extent that there is an incongruity between what is being
affirmed and what is actually happening in the person's life, a kind of
"creative tension" arises in the person's unconscious. This creative tension spurs the unconscious to marshal its vast hidden resources to try to
resolve the incongruity and close the gap, so that the inner and outer realities come into harmony. The unconscious is at work around the clock,
including in sleep, so the seeds of affirmation that are watered every day
can eventually take root and grow in the background of everyday life.

If your partner is using affirmations, you can join in affirming whatever he or she wants by using precisely the same affirmations yourself
on his or her behalf. The process is to first sit down together to draft the
exact language your partner would find most personally meaningful and

reassuring. The affirmations can be for any aspect of health or healing desired. For example, for a heart condition, it might be "My heart is calm, peaceful, and stress-free. My pulse is even and regular. I respond to stress with a deep, relaxing breath." Once the affirmations have been written, you can contribute in two ways:

1. Make a time to sit together and repeat the affirmations. The optimal time would be after meditating together, when you are each in a state of centeredness and peace. In doing this together, the two of you create a shared field of intention that interpenetrates with each of you and amplifies the strength of your individual voices.

2. Practice repeating the affirmations on your own when you are away from your partner, inserting your partner's name (for example, "Helen's heart is calm, peaceful, and stress-free"). In remembering that the two of you are connected—entangled—as two parts of one system that extends over unlimited distance, you can use coaffirmations as a method of distant healing just as you would prayer, Metta, tonglen, or transpersonal imagery.

And, of course, you can add further support by telling your partner when you are going to be practicing these affirmations.

37

Appreciation

OFTEN PATIENTS WHOSE LIVES ARE ABSORBED IN COPING
with a serious illness have lurking in their shadow a hidden sense of
embarrassment or shame, especially if they perceive, rightly or wrongly,
that they are a burden on others. These feelings are subtly encouraged
in a culture that places an exaggerated emphasis on youth, health, and
productivity as sources of personal worth. They can also be triggered by
having an illness that is stigmatizing, poorly understood, or not effectively treated by the patients' doctors. Over time, such feelings can erode
the patients' sense of value and self-esteem, which, of course, can feed
back into poorer coping and adjustment to the illness.

Here is where your expressions of appreciation are especially welcome
and important. If your partner is confronted anew every day with serious
health limitations, you can provide counterassurance every day to prevent or ward off the gremlins of self-doubt. I've seen several couples in
which the well partner spontaneously provides a daily infusion of appreciation. It makes a huge difference to the morale of their partners—they
always notice and are always grateful for it.

To appreciate means literally to *value*. For all the hundreds of studies
that have documented the health effects of social support, it may well be
that it is no more than this simple sense of being valued by others that is
responsible. Expressions of appreciation reinforce a bond and sense of
connection, which, in turn, helps to buffer the effects of stress.

What do you appreciate about your partner? You may be aware of different things at different times. One day it might be a certain personality
attribute, such as a sense of humor. Another day it might be your partner's devotion to you or your family. Another time it might be his or her
perseverance in the face of a seemingly endless chronic illness. And at
times you may be aware of appreciating how the illness has brought the
two of you closer together—what we spoke of earlier as posttraumatic
growth.

PART SEVEN

Simple Gifts

IT'S EASY TO BECOME ABSORBED IN MANAGING THE MORE
formidable challenges of an illness and lose sight of how some very simple strategies can have a surprising impact on your partner's well-being.
Yet often it's the little things that make the biggest difference. Almost
any routine act of daily living can be transformed into a more meaningful
experience by bringing mindfulness and intention to it.

Part 7 offers a mix of "simple gifts"—acts in daily living through which
you can express your caring and offer additional support. We will explore
how such simple gifts as being flexible in your sleeping arrangements,
running a bath for your partner, serving comfort foods or tea, or simply
hanging out with your partner in goal-less togetherness can be real blessings for both of you.

38

Sleeping Separately

ONE OF THE MOST SUPPORTIVE THINGS YOU MAY BE ABLE TO do for you partner is to sleep in another room. There may be initial resistance to this idea from either of you, but it is something you can try to see if it makes a difference in sleep quality for your partner. And it could well be a blessing for you, too.

Sleep and Healing

Many important insights into the quality of sleep have been gained in the last half century. Sleep quality tends to deteriorate naturally with aging for everyone, but people who are ill often have increased sensitivity to disturbance during sleep, and this is particularly problematic because sleep is the time when the body's self-repair mechanisms need to work at their best.

Both psychological and physical well-being are determined in large part by the quality of sleep. The slow-wave (delta) phase is now known to be crucial to tissue repair, and this phase is missing or deficient in many people with chronic illnesses. You know when you've had a night with adequate slow-wave sleep because you awaken feeling refreshed, but when it's been deficient, you awaken feeling exhausted or lethargic. Unfortunately, even though sleep medications may make you sleep for many hours, they are unlikely to correct a deficiency in slow-wave sleep.[1]

The impact of sleep disturbance on the body was recently shown by researchers at Johns Hopkins University School of Medicine. The study involved following thirty-two healthy pain-free women for seven nights. On the first two nights, they slept undisturbed for eight hours. Beginning the third night, they were subjected to either repeated forced awakening or restricted opportunity to sleep (reduced hours), two different ways of cutting their total sleep time in half.

The findings of this experiment were particularly meaningful for partners who are awakened by the other's snoring or restless legs: *interruption of sleep continuity*, rather than the simple reduction in total hours
of sleep, resulted in loss of pain inhibition and increase in spontaneous
pain. "It's not just the total sleep loss, it's the fragmentation," said lead
researcher Michael Smith.[2] This adds to previous studies also showing
that when the slow-wave phase is interrupted, it results in unrefreshing
sleep, diffuse musculoskeletal pain, tenderness, and fatigue in normal
healthy people. Such symptoms are prevalent in people with fibromyalgia and CFS, conditions that are characterized in part by these disturbed
sleep patterns,[3] and also occur in many other conditions. If your partner
has a pain condition of any kind, sleep disturbances may play a role.

On Men and Women

We're also learning more about gender differences in sleep behavior. Sleep is an area that is influenced a great deal by both hormonal
differences between the sexes and age-related differences in circadian
rhythms. Women in middle age are often more sleep-deprived than men
because of hot flashes, general anxieties, or snoring by their male partners. Many suffer in silence rather than move or ask their partner to
sleep elsewhere.

According to sociologist Sara Arber of Sussex University in England,
many couples feel that not sleeping in the same bed is a taboo, but it's really not a reflection on their relationship if they need to sleep separately
to sleep well. In her research, she has found that for most middle-aged
women, eight hours of uninterrupted sleep almost never happens. Many
women find it difficult to fall asleep, wake frequently during the night,
and are then kept awake with worries or by their partner's snoring. Most
men in middle age and older snore, but they snore more loudly than
women. The gender divide seems to be that when women snore, they're
likely to be met with anger from their partner and feel embarrassed for
themselves. When men snore, on the other hand, women tend to greet it
with humor and tolerance.

Arber and her colleagues used surveys and interviews of 1,640 women
and couples and found that both partners often failed to communicate
their needs. She cites the case of a woman who suffered for years with

a husband who would set the alarm at 6:00 A.M., then push the snooze button every five minutes for the next hour. When she finally got up the nerve to tell her husband how this affected her, he was embarrassed and was happy to change his habit.

Arber found that as couples age, their likelihood of sleeping separately increases, with nearly a third doing so after age sixty. She notes that some couples who take the step of sleeping separately report that the quality of their relationship has actually improved as a result.[4]

The bottom line here is that you should talk with your partner frankly about the quality of sleep each of you is getting and whether you want to experiment with sleeping separately. If you can both be reassured that it is not a signal of failure or loss but might actually enhance the quality of your relationship, it may well pay mutual dividends.

39

The Art of the Bath

By preparing a warm bath, Jacuzzi, or hot tub for your partner, you can actually help him or her enjoy the benefits of a remarkably effective healing modality right at home. The use of soaking and bathing is a time-tested remedy in the world's traditions of natural medicine that modern research has found to have many therapeutic benefits. It's also something the two of you can share together if you have a large enough tub.

The Water Cure

Anything that uses water or moisture to stimulate or support the body's healing mechanisms is a form of hydrotherapy. All medical traditions throughout history have used it in some form or another. The healing qualities of water are universally recognized, and hot baths and showers are forms of hydrotherapy appreciated by millions every day.

The modern concept of hydrotherapy as "the water cure" began in Austria in the 1820s and was brought to the United States in 1896 by Benedict Lust, who taught the methods of an Austrian priest named Sebastian Kneipp. Lust had cured himself of tuberculosis using Kneipp's methods and was an enthusiastic advocate of natural therapies. He went on to establish the first American school of naturopathic medicine in New York, and today hydrotherapy is taught in naturopathic medical schools across the United States.

HOW HYDROTHERAPY HELPS

Some methods of hydrotherapy focus on relaxation and some on stimulation. Relaxation comes primarily through the use of warm or hot water, either through soaking or with moving water, as in a Jacuzzi. This is the most common method and the easiest to use for your partner at home.

The main effects are deep relaxation and improved circulation, both of which are profoundly therapeutic for almost any health condition.

Another form that is somewhat more aggressive involves alternating temperature extremes of hot and cold water for purposes of stimulation. In Chinese medicine and Ayurveda, this alternating of extremes is believed to both stimulate and tonify the flow of vital energy (chi, prana) through the body. In naturopathy, it is believed to create a "pumping effect" through the tissues of the body—the heat causes the capillaries to expand, and the cold causes them to contract. When extreme temperatures are alternated at intervals of a few minutes, blood and lymph can be flushed quite efficiently through the body or a specific area.[1]

Any health condition that benefits from improved circulation of energy, blood, and lymph will benefit from a therapeutic bath. Common applications include anxiety and stress reduction, burns, back pain, cancer, chronic obstructive pulmonary disease, skin conditions (such as dermatitis, psoriasis, and scleroderma), detoxification, influenza and the common cold, Crohn's disease, depression, diabetes mellitus, digestive disorders, ear infection, edema, fever, fibromyalgia, headache, heart conditions, inflammation, insomnia, kidney and bladder infections, multiple sclerosis, muscle spasm, musculoskeletal pain, pelvic inflammatory disease, prostatitis, osteoarthritis and rheumatoid arthritis, sprain- and strain-type injuries, sinus infection, varicose veins, and others.

STRATEGIES FOR A BLISSFUL BATH

There are several things you can do to help your partner get the most out of a soak:

- Add bath salts: one half to one pound of Epsom salts added to a bath will aid in relaxing sore muscles and relieving swollen and irritated joints.
- Add essential oils: cedarwood, lemon, rose, orange, and jasmine are all reputed in the naturopathic tradition to have soothing and tranquilizing effects.
- Add valerian as a loose herb for preparing for sleep. (One study found that valerian added to bathwater improved well-being and sleep and reduced pain in fibromyalgia.[2])

- Add chamomile as a loose herb, to soothe the skin and promote sleep.
- Add ginger (sliced or grated) to help relax sore muscles and improve circulation.
- Oatmeal is used to coat, soothe, and restore the skin and is especially good for itchiness, hives, sunburn, and chafing. Put one cup of uncooked oatmeal in a blender, finely blend it, and add it to the bathwater.[3]
- Turn off the lights and use candles.
- Provide a glass of cool, fresh drinking water with a slice of lemon.
- Keep track of the time so your partner doesn't overdo it and end up exhausted or dehydrated.
- Plan the timing so the bath is at least an hour after a not-too-heavy meal.
- Optimal timing is just before bed; lay out a large, soft towel and have the bed ready with fresh, clean sheets.
- Put a glass of fresh drinking water beside the bed for the night.

Finally, consider making this a routine. Repetition of such a relaxing experience has a way of peeling off layers of stress gradually over time. With repetition, your partner's baseline level of tension will steadily diminish and the healing benefits of relaxation will become more apparent.

A FEW WORDS OF CAUTION

In the vast majority of cases, hydrotherapy is safe. However, there are certain conditions in which extremes of heat should not be used and only milder temperatures should be applied. Chief among these are low blood pressure (hypotension), ankylosing spondylitis, and fatigue conditions such as CFS. When immersed for a long time in hot water, some people become dizzy or light-headed upon standing up, so precautions should be taken to avoid falling.

Dehydration can occur as a result of too long a time in hot water. Plenty of drinking water should be available, alcohol should be avoided, and the length of a soak should be limited to prevent both overheating and dehydration. If you or your partner have any concerns about whether hydrotherapy is safe, ask your doctor.

40

Foot Bathing

GIVING YOUR PARTNER A FOOTBATH BRINGS TOGETHER AN interesting mix of health, relational, and even spiritual aspects.

From the point of view of hydrotherapy, a warm footbath is highly therapeutic.[1] The chief benefit is a delightful bodywide relaxation response. Other potential benefits are reducing inflammation or pain in distant areas of the body as well as relieving insomnia, colds, cramps, neuralgia, headaches, shivering, cold hands or feet, nausea, dizziness, or faintness. The key principles are that by drawing greater circulation to the feet, a footbath draws blood and congestion away from distant parts of the body; and the feet have nerve endings and reflex points that help to trigger relaxation throughout the body.

Simply place a tub of warm to hot water on the floor and have your partner sit with his or her feet in water up to the ankles and soak for several minutes. You can use any of the salts, essential oils, or herbs described in the preceding chapter to make it more pleasant.

You can also employ the stimulation principle of hydrotherapy here by using two tubs side by side, one with hot water and one with cold water. Have your partner place his or her feet in the hot water for about three minutes, then move to the cold water for about thirty seconds, then back to the hot for another three minutes, and repeat this sequence a couple of times. This will be a somewhat more stimulating treatment that is also very relaxing.

The ultimate final step is to provide simple massage of your partner's feet afterward with a mild dermatological cream or lotion.

The relational and spiritual symbolism of bathing another's feet adds to the richness of the experience. The origins of foot washing are traced back to ancient civilizations when people primarily wore sandals and their feet were continually exposed to dust and dirt in their environment. Water for people to wash their own feet was offered as an expression of courtesy and hospitality. Religious traditions later began to recognize rich symbolic meaning in humbling oneself to wash another's feet, and it became a gesture of humility for the giver and at the same time a declaration of esteem and spiritual worthiness for the recipient. To give in this way to your partner can be enjoyable for both of you.

41

Food for the Soul

COMFORT FOODS THAT YOU PREPARE FOR YOUR PARTNER
can be a welcome form of support. As you might imagine, what makes
comfort foods comforting is that they help alleviate feelings of distress,
whether from the stress of everyday life or the stress of living with illness
or chronic pain. Certainly there is a strong psychological component
to the satisfaction of having a food that for many years—perhaps since
childhood—has always been associated with good feelings. But beyond
the symbolism of a favorite food in your partner's personal history, there's
also some good science showing that the draw of comfort foods is more
than just psychological.

Researchers at Montclair State University experimented with putting
people in stressful situations and then observed their food choices in
response to the stress. Under stress, people tended to shift their preferences from what we would consider healthful low-fat foods (such as
grapes) to less healthful high-fat or sweet foods (such as M&Ms). They
also found that females were a little more inclined than males to increase
their food consumption in response to stress.[1]

There's a physiological basis for these choices: some of the chemicals
released into the body during the stress response—called glucocorticoids—actually *heighten the sense of pleasure and satisfaction* derived
from eating fatty or sweet foods. In turn, these foods also help to reduce the body's physiological responses to stress.[2] Other studies have
found that foods high in sugar and fat content are more efficient than
healthful foods in reducing negative emotions; conversely, when people are *not* stressed, low-calorie foods are more efficient at increasing
positive emotions.[3] (The downside of this biochemical programming
is that the glucocorticoids that reward comfort eating also increase abdominal fat deposits—hence the links among stress, comfort eating, and
weight gain.)

Needless to say, giving your partner a steady diet of comfort foods may not be a good idea. However, there are times when it might be exactly what is needed to help him or her cope during a difficult stretch. There are certainly some comfort foods that are more healthful than others, and moderation is always possible—especially if accompanied by other comforting strategies such as those described in this book so that food need not become overly important as a source of comfort.

Although you may think you know what your partner would find most comforting, it would be a good idea to ask because you may be surprised. There's some evidence of gender differences in comfort food preferences. For example, at the University of Illinois, Brian Wansink and his colleagues studied such preferences in 1,005 adults and found that while both genders have wide-ranging preferences, males more often preferred warm, hearty, meal-related comfort foods (such as steak, casseroles, and soups), whereas females more often preferred those that were snack-related (such as chocolate and ice cream). There was also evidence of differences by age: younger people often have a stronger preference for snack-related items than do those in their fifties and older.[4]

Almost anything can serve the function of a comfort food, and there are obviously many more kinds of comfort foods than can be mentioned here. To get a sense of types of comfort foods that are most popular, I took an informal poll of couples in my projects and found a few broad categories, as described below.

Hot Dishes

By far the most commonly mentioned comfort foods were those that could be described as warm, thick, and hearty. The favorite among these was macaroni and cheese, followed by poached eggs on toast, oatmeal, porridge, and potato dishes—scalloped or mashed. Then there were the gravy dishes, over either potatoes or meatballs. Also in this category were meat loaf, steamed pork dumplings, casserole dishes, and shepherd's pie. Of course, pasta dishes of all kinds can deliver real comfort—favorites were linguini and clams, scallops, and shrimp over pasta. Then there were more complex offerings like lobster bisque, seafood quiche, eggs Benedict, and haddock Florentine. A popular complement to many of the above were heated breads, especially in the form of toast, warm bagels, or dinner rolls.

Soups

The next most mentioned category of comfort foods was soups. A publishing empire has been built on the metaphor of one of the most popular comfort foods—chicken soup—and certainly chicken is a key ingredient in countless varieties of soups for comfort. It seems to offer a universally pleasing combination of texture and taste. Nevertheless, there are other kinds of soup that can be comforting as well. Chief among these are soups that offer texture or thickness: lentil soups and chowders (corn, clam) are favorites, as are chili, kale soup with kielbasa, French onion soup, and rice congee.

Fruit-Based Snacks

I was surprised to see how many people regard fruit and nut-based dishes as comfort foods. Several reported their favorites were freshly picked berries with cream or whipped cream, and a few added fresh hot scones or shortcake to the mix. Others liked cooked or stewed fruits such as pears or apples (cooking brings out the sugars), again with cream or whipped cream and perhaps a dash of cinnamon. Instead of whipped cream, some preferred frozen yogurt or even ice cream with their fruit. You can easily add your partner's favorite nuts (chopped for finer texture) to any of the above to round out the taste/texture experience.

Of course, the fruit smoothie has become a favorite by virtue of its combination of texture, smoothness, thickness, and sweetness.

Cool and Creamy

In addition to the fruit smoothie, several other forms of cool or cold and creamy foods were popular sources of comfort. These included all puddings, custards, yogurts, frozen yogurts, and ice creams. Plain yogurt can be dressed up with little effort to be surprisingly comforting and healthful at the same time. Consider, for example, the virtues of an organic fat-free yogurt with just a little honey or maple syrup added. As an alternative sweetener, just a few drops of the concentrated herbal sweetener stevia can substitute for the honey or maple syrup.

Tapioca pudding has some unique textural qualities. And some rather creative versions of ice cream are now available, offering the opportunity for your partner to have almost any favorite flavor (garlic ice cream is a perennial favorite at the annual garlic festival in Gilroy, California).

Other Preparations

Foods that offer contrasts of temperature or texture were also reported as favorites. A few examples include warm apple pie à la mode, fresh-baked chocolate chip cookies dunked in milk, or a hot-fudge brownie sundae (my personal favorite). Then there are taste contrasts: some people like to combine sweet and salty tastes for comfort—such as Brenda, who prefers a cocktail of potato chips and chocolate.

Honorable mention should certainly go to grilled cheese sandwiches, rice pudding, bread pudding, bread chunks soaked in milk with a little sugar and cinnamon, graham crackers and milk, and hot cinnamon rolls.

A Special Case: Chocolate

Special attention is in order here for one of the most important—and possibly most healthful—comfort foods, chocolate. There is a long history of chocolate's being used for medicinal purposes. In a review of the literature on medicinal uses of chocolate, Dr. Teresa Dillinger of the Department of Nutrition at the University of California, Davis, found an amazing array of uses throughout history. Conditions treated have included fatigue, fever and panting of breath, faintness of heart, emaciation, anemia, poor appetite, mental fatigue, poor breast milk production, consumption/tuberculosis, fever, gout, kidney stones, and poor sexual appetite/low virility. Other applications include stimulating the nervous system, improving digestion and elimination, stimulating the kidneys, promoting longevity, and improving bowel function. Chocolate paste has also been used as a carrier to administer drugs.[5]

Recent studies have confirmed that chocolate can indeed have therapeutic effects. Chief among these studies are those indicating benefits for blood pressure and cardiovascular risk factors. For example, researchers at a primary care clinic in Germany compared the effects of high-quality dark chocolate to white chocolate in people with high blood pressure. After eighteen weeks, those taking dark chocolate had significantly reduced blood pressure (both systolic and diastolic) without changes in body weight, plasma levels of lipids, glucose, or free radicals in the blood. The prevalence of hypertension declined from 86 percent to 68 percent in this group, but none of these beneficial changes were seen in those taking white chocolate.[6] Another study with hypertension patients found that dark chocolate decreased blood pressure and serum LDL (low-density lipoprotein) cholesterol and improved dilation of blood vessels.[7]

It seems that the key beneficial ingredient in chocolate is its content of polyphenol (a plant substance with antioxidant qualities). Polyphenols are particularly high in dark chocolate but absent in white chocolate and have been found in numerous studies to contribute to reduced risk of heart disease, cancer, and strokes. Dark chocolate reduces factors that promote LDL (bad) cholesterol, and increases antioxidant capacity and concentration of HDL (good) cholesterol in the blood, without adversely affecting prostaglandins (important hormones that regulate a variety of important bodily functions).[8] It is rich in flavonoids (antioxidants), improves functioning of the cells that line the blood vessels (endothelial cells), and is associated with an increase in blood levels of epicatechin, which improves blood flow.[9] It also increases insulin sensitivity, which serves a good antidiabetes function.[10]

As for cancer, there's laboratory evidence suggesting that ingredients in chocolate inhibit the growth of prostate and breast cancer cells, although there have been no studies of people using chocolate as an anticancer treatment.[11] But in chronic fatigue syndrome, a recent study at the Hull Royal Infirmary in the United Kingdom found that people with CFS who ingested forty-five grams (about an ounce and a half) of high-quality dark chocolate (85 percent cocoa) each day for eight weeks had significantly reduced symptoms, without weight gain, compared to another eight-week period in which they took a simulated dark chocolate.[12]

Is chocolate the ultimate comfort food? That's a matter of personal taste, but it may be among the most healthful. In any case, you have to be careful in distinguishing among the many forms of it on the market. The studies showing health benefits all used a high-quality dark chocolate (70 percent or more cocoa) in relatively small amounts. This is very different from the most readily available forms of chocolate candy, which tend to have a low concentration of cocoa coupled with a high concentration of sugar and fat. A chocolate product's cocoa percentage is usually listed in the ingredients, and you can find high-quality dark chocolate in health food stores and some gourmet specialty shops. You can do your partner a favor by being discriminating in your choice of chocolate; with higher quality, less is more.

Comfort Food Recipes

Of course there are innumerable cookbooks out there. Here are a few good ones that offer easy and delicious recipes for comfort foods: *The Food You Crave: Luscious Recipes for a Healthy Life* by Ellie Krieger, *The New Moosewood Cookbook* by Mollie Katzen, *The Art of Simple Food* by Alice Waters, and *Quick Vegetarian Pleasures* by Jeanne Lemlin. In addition, www.epicurious.com and www.foodnetwork.com are good websites for finding recipes to make just about anything.

42

The Art of Tea

THE PREPARATION OF HERBAL AND MEDICINAL TEAS IS AN
ancient healing practice rich in symbolism yet often overlooked in modern times as a source of comfort in illness. When you provide a refreshing cup of tea to your partner, you are offering many benefits. Serving tea is really a holistic therapy in the sense that it is good for mind, body, and spirit, as well as your relationship.

Choices of Tea

Certain teas have some noteworthy medicinal effects that have been well documented. The two most common types of tea, green and black, both come from the same plant (*Camellia sinensis*). Green tea is produced by lightly steaming the freshly cut leaves, while black tea is produced by allowing the leaves to oxidize. During this oxidation for black tea, enzymes present in the tea leaves reduce the strength of many therapeutic substances, making them much less active.

With green tea, oxidation is not allowed to take place because the steaming process inactivates these enzymes. Thus, green tea remains very high in polyphenols, which have potent antioxidant and anticancer properties.[1] Both green and black teas have other substances that promote cardiovascular health, may help reduce stress, and may reduce cholesterol levels.[2] Unfortunately for black tea lovers, however, there is a caveat: milk counteracts the beneficial effects of tea on cardiovascular health, because the casein protein contained in milk actually eliminates the beneficial substances from the tea that confer the cardio-protective effect. Thus, if maximum health benefit is what you're after, black tea should be served without milk.[3]

While green and black are the most studied types of tea, there are many other kinds that may confer health benefits as well that don't have the benefit of as much scientific scrutiny. In fact, any herb can be consumed as a tea, and there are hundreds of medicinal herbs. If your partner is so inclined, you could explore the landscape of medicinal teas together (try Googling tea for any specific symptom and you'll find many options) or consult with an herbalist. The traditions of Oriental medicine (Chinese medicine and Ayurveda) offer a whole panoply of tea recommendations based on the subtle energetic qualities of herbs matched to the unique needs of the recipient. The Western naturopathic tradition as well has a huge array of herbal tea recommendations based on specific symptoms and ailments.

In terms of scientific evidence, you can't beat green tea as a broad-spectrum remedy. Just sweeten with a little honey, sugar, or stevia. However, your partner may have another favorite or may wish to experiment with a variety of teas, and there's no reason not to.

A Healing Ritual

Many volumes have been written about the therapeutic benefits of drinking a cup of tea, but before any medicinal effects take place, consider the experience itself. Since preparing a cup of tea for your partner begins with an intention to serve, it's an opportunity for you to be in a giving state of mind and access your heart. Let the preparation become a thoughtful ritual into which you channel compassionate intention throughout the process. Let the whole experience be one of mindfulness: rather than rushing through (or using the microwave), take your time and be as present as you can for the full experience of each step.

1. Prepare the kettle by emptying it of old water.
2. Put fresh water (filtered if possible[4]) in the kettle.
3. Wait for the water to boil, letting this be a time of patience: enjoy this special gap in time, letting it be a "waiting meditation" or simply resting as nature takes its course with the water.
4. Gather the tea, being mindful as you open the box and take the tea bag or as you place the loose tea into the infuser.
5. Place the tea bag or infuser in the cup carefully rather than just plopping it in.
6. Pour in the water slowly and with as much presence as you can.

7. Carry this gift to your partner, thinking of it as a love offering and delivering it with a smile.
8. Sit down with your partner and sip tea quietly and mindfully together.

Anytime your partner is in distress, a cup of his or her favorite tea may help simply by virtue of the "pattern interrupt" that it induces through relaxation and attention to the moment. Having tea is an experience that naturally leads to relaxation, which is, of course, one of the body's most healing states. It's hard to gulp tea down; it's much easier to sip it slowly, and doing so tends to slow us down and encourage relaxation. In fact, it's hard not to sip mindfully—you have to really pay attention to do it—so it's a natural experience of meditation.

Perhaps your partner has a favorite cup to be used for tea. Using the same favorite cup helps to ritualize the experience. The cup then becomes a cue that can help trigger the state of relaxation that it has brought so many times before. You might consider other items such as saucers or tray tables that can also, in time, become consistent cues for feelings of relaxation and comfort.

While there's considerable research on medicinal uses of tea, it's debatable how much the therapeutic benefits are due to the botanical qualities of specific teas versus the wonderful mind-body relaxation effects induced by the experience of sipping tea. If your partner is suffering from a particular illness for which a certain kind of tea has been reported to have medicinal effects, be careful about imposing this on him or her. It may be far more therapeutic to serve your partner's favorite tea that reinforces comfort and good feelings than to forsake this personal pleasure for a strange new "clinically correct" tea.

43

Simple Pleasures

WITH THIS CHAPTER, I ENCOURAGE YOU TO TAKE SOME TIME together for simple pleasures. For many couples living with illness, it's easy to become so absorbed in the challenges of health or attending to medical treatments that you lose track of your connection with each other. This is when it's good to take a break—a "pattern interrupt"—from coping, striving, and surviving and simply have some quiet time in goal-less togetherness. This can also help to reaffirm that you are more than your body and that life is bigger than physical health alone.

I have assembled below some descriptions from several couples of how they have maintained simple pleasures over time in their relationship, despite health challenges and other crises. I invite you to read between the lines and see what it is that is being affirmed in each of these accounts.

My husband and I just celebrated our thirty-ninth wedding anniversary. The one thing that we have done for simple pleasure and continue to do is play cards (though once in a while we play dominoes). Most of the time the game is rummy. We play when we can and may also use some of this time to discuss issues and make plans. What makes this game unique for us is that we have a log of the results that is kept in a bound journal. We started it in 1984. My husband has an incredible winning record because, while playing, I have a tendency to wander mentally. Of course, he knows that and takes advantage of me during those times. It is such a pleasure to review the scores, the drawings, and the comments in the journal. We will continue the log and will forever have the documented scores to cherish.

✦ ✦ ✦

We have a screened-in porch with soft, glowing string lights across the ceiling—red on one side and green on the other, like the port and starboard sides of a sailboat. We turn all our lights off except the string lights and have candles on the porch table. We have two comfortable porch chairs side by side, and we share a footstool. We face out and watch the fireflies blinking and dancing in patterns on the lawn. It is just peaceful sitting there together enjoying the sounds of nature and watching the little lights blink here and there. Sometimes we watch the moon coming up over the water.

Our porch roof has skylights, so on clear nights sometimes we lay the backs of our lounge chairs down, side by side, so we can recline and watch the stars. Other times it's nice to sit and watch and listen to the rain, then watch the rainbow come out after the rain.

In our living room, we have LED string lights around the top of the walls near the ceiling. They give off a warm glow, and we turn all the other lights off and sit side by side on the couch and share a footstool, listening to soft music together.

, , ,

We like walking on the beach at sunset. There are very few people at that time of day, the temperature is cool after a hot day, and the view is spectacular [on the Maine coast]. We may also bundle up and walk during early fall or late spring when the weather permits.

, , ,

We simply like to spend time together; it doesn't matter what we're doing. Sometimes it's a walk or just sitting outside reading individually or kayaking together. . . . Sometimes he'll fish and I'll just read. I guess the key here is simple togetherness.

, , ,

My husband and I love to take a walk together with our dog on one of the many great walking trails nearby. . . . We have the trail map and like to explore a new trail together. He's very understanding if my energy is low and I have to stop to rest or stop altogether.

, , ,

I would say that our simple pleasure is having someone watch the kids while we order Chinese takeout, rent a movie, and eat while watching the movie in bed, where we can feel connected, kidless, and young.

❯ ❯ ❯

We enjoy brook trout fishing. We have a small, lightweight canoe that we can paddle easily in small ponds and streams. We travel two or three hours for a pleasant ride and then enjoy the peace and pleasure of a remote location, seeing animals in the wild, and catching (often releasing) brook trout.

❯ ❯ ❯

Our simple pleasure is a day at the seaside. We like sun, sand, and sea. A bag of tokens for the amusement slot machines, a game of crazy golf, and fish-and-chips for our dinner. If there's a brass band playing somewhere and a few deck chairs available, all the better.

❯ ❯ ❯

Our simple pleasure started thirteen years ago when we were dating. Every Sunday we sit together and do the *Boston Globe Magazine* crossword puzzle. Although we now have two young children, we still try to sit on Sunday evenings to do the puzzle.

❯ ❯ ❯

We discovered *CSI: Las Vegas* while I was going through chemo, and we would look forward to watching it together almost every night, as we had seen none of the series. It was interesting and engaging and made me forget any discomfort I might be experiencing.

❯ ❯ ❯

I love it when my husband gives me a gentle back rub. Yes, it relieves my pain for a while. I particularly like to get in the hot tub with him to just relax, not to speak, but to enjoy the sounds of nature and totally relax. I love the hot tub and listening to the birds and waiting for the sun to set. It is a great way to end the day. Also it's a good time for me to get in touch with my spiritual side.

I particularly enjoy sitting with my husband in some deep-cushioned outdoor furniture that I recently purchased, and reading or napping. Just sitting quietly and watching the world go by—it is very relaxing.

Another simple pleasure that I absolutely love is to go down to take off our shoes and walk on the beach for an hour or so. Not running or jogging, just holding hands and walking at a comfortable pace. This is also a wonderful way to end a hectic workday—or a great treat for a weekend.

We have bird feeders in the backyard, and I *love* to watch the birds and see the babies coming to the feeder and watch the interaction between the parents and babies. How the mother and father birds will actually show the babies how to eat out of the feeder. Nature is amazing.

➤   ➤   ➤

We love to light a fire, turn the lights down low (even off), light some candles—they should be scattered all over the room—and listen to music (you have to have a CD player that allows you to skip particular songs, crank up other songs, switch the mood as your mind's mood switches and jumps). There is no need for talking. Sometimes—well, actually, often—I find lyrics have captured my emotions better than I can ever articulate them.

➤   ➤   ➤

My husband and I like to watch a movie at home. It seems to be relaxing, and we both enjoy the movies. We also enjoy going for walks together.

➤   ➤   ➤

My favorite simple pleasure that I share with my spouse is Sunday morning—coffee and newspaper. We have a small love seat that holds only two, and it's set by the window in a really sunny corner. I usually wake up later to the smell of coffee brewing and the paper waiting for me. We sit together for at least an hour just reading and chatting.

➤   ➤   ➤

We like to take walks together in the evening with no destination in particular and hold hands. The hand holding is key, for we came to each other later in life and never got to go to the dance. It is an affirmation of our connectedness. We also like to go to the ocean's rocky shore and just sit, watching the endless, graceful motion of the water. The power and beauty of the shifting color and constant movement brings us to a quieter place within.

❧ ❧ ❧

We have three dogs, and we walk them together around the neighborhood. We occasionally take them to the beach or on a trail along a large stream so the dogs can go swimming.

❧ ❧ ❧

Simple pleasures together—walking, bike riding, hiking, skiing, sitting out front just about any time of day, working in the garden, listening to music, being with our kids most of the time.

❧ ❧ ❧

One of our simple pleasures is yawning. Just to feel better, we like to try yawning five or six times in a row. It is easy to induce and very contagious between two people. Best results are yawning with an audible sigh on the exhale.

Epilogue

HEALING MEANS MORE THAN JUST MEDICAL RECOVERY. IT means becoming more whole and complete as a human being. Any healing that occurs anywhere along the entire continuum of body, mind, spirit, and relationships makes us more whole. In remembering this, some form of healing is always possible for anyone no matter what is going on medically; even in a dying process, there is abundant opportunity for healing to occur.

This book has been about how you can support healing in a loved one on whatever level might be possible. In expressing your caring through the ways described, or any other ways, you become more whole yourself. You are more in touch with your heart, the two of you have a deeper connection with one another and the bond becomes stronger. It is my hope that partners everywhere will claim their true potential as healers in this way.

DVD Program
Touch, Caring and Cancer

MANY OF THE TECHNIQUES DESCRIBED IN PART 3 ARE TAUGHT in the award-winning[1] DVD program *Touch, Caring and Cancer: Simple Instruction for Family and Friends,* published by Collinge and Associates. This is a complete program that provides detailed instruction by leading experts in oncology massage for safe and simple techniques that anyone can learn and apply for the comfort of a cancer patient. Developed as part of the author's NCI-sponsored research, it follows eleven patients and their care partners through a workshop as they receive hands-on instruction and practice the techniques together.

The DVD runs seventy-eight minutes and is accompanied by an illustrated manual. Chapters include: Introduction, Safety Precautions, Positioning, Communication, Frame of Mind, Centering, The Head and Face, The Neck, Shoulders and Back, The Hands, The Feet, Acupressure, and Closing Thoughts.

Contributors to the program include William Collinge, PhD, project director; Janet Kahn, PhD, NCTMB, University of Vermont College of Medicine and advisor to NIH on complementary and alternative medicine; Tracy Walton, MS, LMT, national trainer in oncology massage and co-investigator in NCI-sponsored research; David Rosenthal, MD, Dana-Farber/Harvard Cancer Center and former president of the American Cancer Society; and Susan Bauer-Wu, PhD, RN, Distinguished Cancer Scholar, Emory University, and NCI-sponsored researcher.

The program is available in English, Spanish, and Chinese versions. For more information visit www.PartnersinHealing.net.

Additional Resources

Training Opportunities in Energy Healing Techniques

Instruction in energy healing can come in a couple of ways. One is to seek an organized training experience in the form of a workshop or seminar, such as through one of the organizations listed below. The alternative is to seek direct instruction from a local practitioner who is willing to work with you and your partner privately to teach basic techniques pertinent to your unique situation. Often just a little direct instruction is enough to grasp some basic skills, but if you can attend a workshop you will probably receive a more complete understanding. The two most widely available forms of instruction are in Healing Touch and Reiki.

HEALING TOUCH

The Healing Touch Program is the official organization that provides training in Healing Touch, which incorporates many of the techniques described in part 4: Simple Energy Healing Practices. Both laypeople and health professionals are welcome to receive their training. There are several levels of training leading to certification, but the first level alone is sufficient to gain a good understanding of the basics you can start with for family and friends. Training is usually conducted in the form of one- or two-day workshops, which are conducted in many cities across the United States and internationally. A listing of workshops and teachers is posted on the website below.

For more information see www.healingtouchprogram.com

REIKI

One of the more accessible forms of energy healing in most communities is Reiki. There are many organizations and thousands of practitioners and teachers, making this the most widely available modality of energy healing. The easiest way to find out about instruction locally is to go onto the internet and google "Reiki" followed by the name of your town or city, and you are likely to see a list of practitioners who can inform you about learning opportunities in your area. As with the Healing Touch Program, training in Reiki usually takes place in the form of one- or two-day workshops. The two leading organizations in the United States are the Reiki Alliance and the International Association of Reiki Professionals, both of whose websites are listed below. Another useful website is Holistic WebWorks, which provides a comprehensive listing of Reiki organizations worldwide. For more information visit the following websites:

> The Reiki Alliance: www.reikialliance.com
> Inaternational Association of Reiki Professionals: www.iarp.org
> Holistic Webworks: www.holisticwebworks.com/Reiki-Associations.htm

Organizations Providing Information and Support for Caregivers

AMERICAN CANCER SOCIETY

The American Cancer Society is the largest information and support organization for cancer, with local offices in most communities. Their programs include include both online and local education and support offerings for patients, caregivers, and sometimes couples. For more information see www.cancer.org.

AMERICAN HEART ASSOCIATION

The American Heart Association has a website with an abundance of information about caregiving for people with heart and stroke-related conditions. The site also provides online discussion groups and links for information about local support groups, including some for caregivers. For more information see www.americanheart.org.

CANCERCARE, INC.

CancerCare, Inc., is a national nonprofit organization that provides free, professional support services over the phone for anyone affected by cancer, including family members. Their website provides free support groups for caregivers both online and by telephone. For more information see www.cancercare.org.

CAREGIVER.COM

CareGiver.com is a leading provider of support and information for caregivers of all types. The website includes a database listing local support groups. There are individual channels on the site pertaining to Alzheimer's disease, bipolar disorder, caregiver stories, long-term care, medication management, mobility limitations, ovarian cancer, rural caregivers, schizophrenia, and technology for caregiving. For more information see www.caregiver.com.

COLLINGE AND ASSOCIATES

Collinge and Associates conducts research and provides consultation and educational programs in the fields of complementary therapies and caregiving. The website contains writings by William Collinge on topics in integrative health care, summaries of his research studies in complementary therapies and caregiving, excerpts from his books, announcements of workshops and retreats, and information about CD audio programs and the DVD program *Touch, Caring and Cancer: Simple Instruction for Family and Friends*. For more information see www.collinge.org.

FAMILY CAREGIVER ALLIANCE

Family Caregiver Alliance offers programs at national, state, and local levels. Their website conducts online support groups for caregivers of adults with disorders such as Alzheimer's, stroke, brain injury, and other chronic debilitating health conditions; caregivers of people with Huntington's disease and movement disorders; lesbian, gay, bisexual, and transgender caregivers of adults with chronic health problems; and clients of California's Caregiver Resource Centers. For more information see www.caregiver.org.

NATIONAL ALLIANCE FOR CAREGIVING

The National Alliance for Caregiving is a nonprofit coalition of national organizations focusing on issues of family caregiving. Alliance members include grassroots organizations, professional associations, service organizations, disease-specific organizations, a government agency, and corporations. Their website provides educational materials for caregivers, national statistics on caregiving, and reviews and ratings of over a thousand books, videos, websites, and training materials on caregiving. For more information see www.caregiving.org.

NATIONAL FAMILY CAREGIVERS ASSOCIATION (NFCA)

The NFCA site provides caregivers with tips and advocacy updates, as well as information on communicating effectively with healthcare professionals. The site also offers a section on sharing your caregiving story, where family caregivers can write in to share their personal caregiving experience. Additionally, the site provides information on becoming an NFCA member and ordering publications. For more information see www.thefamilycaregiver.org.

THE WELLNESS COMMUNITY

The Wellness Community is a national organization with chapters in many major cities that offer support programs for both patients and family members, primarily dealing with cancer but sometimes related to other illnesses as well. For more information see www.thewellnesscom munity.org.

THE WELL SPOUSE ASSOCIATION

Well Spouse is a national, not-for-profit membership organization that gives support to wives, husbands, and partners of the chronically ill or disabled. The website contains a listing of local member support groups around the United States, as well as descriptions of the following organizational offerings: the newsletter *Mainstay*, an online mentorship program for members to receive guidance in how to support other caregivers; letter-writing groups for caregiver support; respite weekends; an online forum for spousal caregivers; and a one-day workshop (Caregiver Journey) presented across the country by local members. For more information see www.wellspouse.org.

Notes

Introduction

1. National Cancer Institute, http://seer.cancer.gov/statfacts/html/all.html.
2. L. E. Fields, V. L. Burt, J. A. Cutler, J. Hughes, E. J. Roccella, P. Sorlie. "The Burden of Adult Hypertension in the United States 1999 to 2000: A Rising Tide." *Hypertension* 44, no. 4 (Oct. 2004): 398–404.
3. R. M. Gallagher. "Headache Pain." *Journal of the American Osteopathic Association* 105, no. 9, Supplement 4 (Sept. 2005): S7–11.
4. Centers for Disease Control and Prevention (CDC). State prevalence of self-reported doctor-diagnosed arthritis and arthritis-attributable activity limitation—United States, 2003. *Morbidity and Mortality Weekly Report* 55, no. 17 (May 2006): 477–81.
5. American Heart Association, www.americanheart.org.
6. A. A. Ginde, K. E. Delaney, R. M. Lieberman, S. G. Vanderweil, C. A. Camargo Jr. "Estimated Risk for Undiagnosed Diabetes in the Emergency Department: A Multicenter Survey." *Academic and Emergency Medicine* 14, no. 5 (May 2007): 492–95.
7. T. W. Strine, J. M. Hootman. "U.S. National Prevalence and Correlates of Low Back and Neck Pain among Adults." *Arthritis and Rheumatism* 57, no. 4 (May 2007): 656–65.
8. Alzheimer's Association, www.alz.org.
9. American College of Rheumatology. www.rheumatology.org/public/factsheets/fibromya_new.asp? Accessed 12/1/07.
10. Centers for Disease Control and Prevention (CDC), www.cdc.gov/cfs/cfsbasicfacts.htm.
11. C. Bouchardy, G. Fioretta, H. M. Verkooijen, G. Vlastos, P. Schaefer, J. F. Delaloye, I. Neyroud-Caspar, S. Balmer Majno, Y. Wespi, M. Forni, P. Chappuis, A. P. Sappino, E. Rapiti. "Recent Increase of Breast Cancer Incidence among Women under the Age of Forty." *British Journal of Cancer* 96, no. 11 (June 2007): 1743–46.
12. A. G. Mainous III, V. A. Diaz, C. J. Everett. "Assessing Risk for Development of Diabetes in Young Adults." *Annals of Family Medicine* 5, no. 5 (Sept.–Oct. 2007): 425–29.
13. R. W. Jeffery, N. E. Sherwood. "Is the Obesity Epidemic Exaggerated? No." *British Medical Journal* 336, no. 7638 (Feb. 2008): 245.

14. R. M. Eraso, N. J. Bradford, C. N. Fontenot, L. R. Espinoza, A. Gedalia. "Fibromyalgia Syndrome in Young Children: Onset at Age 10 Years and Younger." *Clinical and Experimental Rheumatology* 25, no. 4 (July–Aug. 2007): 639–44; H. Knoop, M. Stulemeijer, L. W. de Jong, T. J. Fiselier, G. Bleijenberg. "Efficacy of Cognitive Behavioral Therapy for Adolescents with Chronic Fatigue Syndrome: Long-term Follow-up of a Randomized, Controlled Trial." *Pediatrics* 121, no. 3 (Mar. 2008): e619–25.

15. Ayya Khema, *When the Iron Eagle Flies: Buddhism for the West* (New York: Penguin, 1991).

16. O. Kravdal, "The Impact of Marital Status on Cancer Survival," *Social Service and Medicine* 52, no. 3 (Feb. 2001): 357–68.

17. A. Ikeda, H. Iso, H. Toyoshima, Y. Fujino, T. Mizoue, T. Yoshimura, Y. Inaba, and A. Tamakoshi—JACC Study Group, "Marital Status and Mortality among Japanese Men and Women: The Japan Collaborative Cohort Study," *BMC Public Health* 7 (May 7, 2007): 73.

18. S. Ebrahim, G. Wannamethee, A. McCallum, M. Walker, and A. G. Shaper, "Marital Status, Change in Marital Status, and Mortality in Middle-Aged British Men," *American Journal of Epidemiology* 142, no. 8 (Oct. 15, 1995): 834–42.

19. National Family Caregivers Association. NFCA Caregiver Survey, July 2000. www.nfcacares.org/who_are_family_caregivers/2000_survey.cfm.

20. R. McCorkle and J. V. Pasacreta, "Enhancing Caregiver Outcomes in Palliative Care," *Cancer Control* 8, no. 1 (2001): 36–45; J. Ross, "A Looming Public Health Crisis: The Nursing Shortage of Today," *Journal of Perianesthesia Nursing* 17, no. 5 (2002): 337–40; J. Harden, A. Schafenacker, L. Northouse, D. Mood, D. Smith, K. Pienta, M. Hussain, and K. Baranowski, "Couples' Experiences with Prostate Cancer: Focus Group Research," *Oncology Nursing Forum* 29, no. 4 (2002): 701–9.

21. W. Collinge, J. Kahn, P. Yarnold, R. McCorkle, and S. Bauer-Wu, "Couples and Cancer: Feasibility of Brief Instruction in Massage and Touch Therapy to Build Caregiver Efficacy," *Journal of the Society for Integrative Oncology* 5, no. 4 (2007): 147–54.

22. J. L. Wolff, S. M. Dy, K. D. Frick, and J. D. Kasper, "End-of-Life Care: Findings from a National Survey of Informal Caregivers," *Archives of Internal Medicine* 167, no. 1 (Jan. 8, 2007): 40–46.

23. B. R. Cassileth and A. J. Vickers, "Massage Therapy for Symptom Control: Outcome Study at a Major Cancer Center," *Journal of Pain and Symptom Management* 28, no. 3 (2004): 244–49.

24. "Promoting Healthy Aging through 'Elder-Healer' Training," grant 43AG24016-01 (2004), William Collinge, principal investigator, National Institute on Aging, National Institutes of Health.

25. R. McCorkle and J. Pasacreta, "Enhancing Caregiver Outcomes in Palliative Care," *Cancer Control* 8, no. 1 (2001): 36–45.

26. J. V. Pasacreta, F. Barg, I. Nuamah, and R. McCorkle, "Participant Characteristics before and 4 Months after Attendance at a Family Caregiver Cancer Education Program," *Cancer Nursing* 23, no. 4 (2000): 295–303.

27. T. Field, M. Hernandez-Reif, O. Quintino, et al., "Elder Retired Volunteers Benefit from Giving Massage Therapy to Infants," *Journal of Applied Gerontology* 17 (1997): 229–39.

1. The Paradox of Caring

1. D. K. Wellisch, K. R. Jamison, and R. O. Passau, "Psychosocial Aspects of Mastectomy II: The Man's Perspective," *American Journal of Psychiatry* 135 (1978): 543–46; M. Keller, G. Henrich, M. Beutel, et al., "Mutuality of Distress and Support in Couples Including a Cancer Patient," *Psychotherapy, Psychoanalytics and Medical Psychology* 48, nos. 9–10 (1998): 358–68; M. Omne-Ponte, L. Homnber, R. Bergstron, et al., "Psychosocial Adjustment among Husbands of Women Treated for Breast Cancer: Mastectomy versus Breast Conserving Surgery," *European Journal of Cancer* 29A (1993): 1393–97; L. L. Northouse, D. Mood, T. Templin, et al., "Couples' Patterns of Adjustment to Colon Cancer," *Social Science and Medicine* 50, no. 2 (2000): 271–84; L. Baider and A. DeNour, "Couples' Reactions and Adjustment to Mastectomy: A Preliminary Report," *International Journal of Psychiatry in Medicine* 14 (1984): 265–76; L. Baider and A. Kaplan De-Nour, "Adjustment to Cancer: Who Is the Patient—The Husband or the Wife?" *Israeli Journal of Medical Science* 24, nos. 9–10 (1988): 631–36; R. Kirschner-Hermanns and G. Jakse, "Quality of Life Following Radical Prostatectomy," *Critical Reviews of Oncology and Hematology* 43, no. 2 (2002): 141.

2. A. Bandura, *Self-Efficacy: The Exercise of Control* (New York: Freeman, 1997); A. Bandura, "Self-Efficacy: Toward a Unifying Theory of Behavioral Change," *Psychological Review* 84 (1977): 191–215; C. C. Benight and A. Bandura, "Social Cognitive Theory of Posttraumatic Recovery: The Role of Perceived Self-Efficacy," *Behavioral Research and Therapy* 42, no. 10 (Oct. 2004): 1129–48; A. Bandura, L. Reese, and N. E. Adams, "Micro-Analysis of Action and Fear Arousal as a Function of Differential Levels of Perceived Self-Efficacy," *Journal of Personality and Social Psychology* 43 (1982): 5–21; A. Bandura, C. B. Taylor, S. L. Williams, et al., "Catecholamine Secretion as a Function of Perceived Coping Self-Efficacy," *Journal of Consulting and Clinical Psychology* 53 (1985): 406–14.

3. J. L. Cameron, R. L. Franche, A. M. Cheung, and D. E. Stewart, "Lifestyle Interference and Emotional Distress in Family Caregivers of Advanced Cancer Patients," *Cancer* 94, no. 2 (2002): 521–27.

4. W. E. Haley, L. A. LaMonde, B. Han, S. Narramore, and R. Schonwetter, "Family Caregiving in Hospice: Effects on Psychological and Health Functioning

among Spousal Caregivers of Hospice Patients with Lung Cancer or Dementia," *Hospital Journal* 15, no. 4 (2001): 1–18.

5. R. Glaser, J. Sheridan, W. B. Malarkey, R. C. MacCallum, and J. K. Kiecolt-Glaser, "Chronic Stress Modulates the Immune Response to a Pneumococcal Pneumonia Vaccine," *Psychosomatic Medicine* 62, no. 6 (2000): 804–7.

6. Michelle M. Bishop, Jennifer L. Beaumont, Elizabeth A. Hahn, David Cella, Michael A. Andrykowski, Marianne J. Brady, Mary M. Horowitz, Kathleen A. Sobocinski, J. Douglas Rizzo, and John R. Wingard, "Late Effects of Cancer and Hematopoietic Stem-Cell Transplantation on Spouses or Partners Compared with Survivors and Survivor-Matched Controls," *Journal of Clinical Oncology* 25, no. 11 (Apr. 10, 2007): 1403–11.

7. L. Northouse, T. Templin, and D. Mood, "Couples' Adjustment to Breast Disease during the First Year Following Diagnosis," *Journal of Behavioral Medicine* 24, no. 2 (2001): 115–36.

8. M. J. Rohrbaugh, V. Shoham, J. C. Coyne, J. A. Cranford, J. S. Sonnega, and J. M. Nicklas, "Beyond the 'Self' in Self-Efficacy: Spouse Confidence Predicts Patient Survival Following Heart Failure," *Journal of Family Psychology* 18, no. 1 (Mar. 2004): 184–93.

9. H. Soubhi, M. Fortin, and C. Hudon, "Perceived Conflict in the Couple and Chronic Illness Management: Preliminary Analyses from the Quebec Health Survey," *BMC Family Practice* 7 (Oct. 19, 2006): 59.

10. M. J. Rohrbaugh, V. Shoham, and J. C. Coyne, "Effect of Marital Quality on Eight-Year Survival of Patients with Heart Failure," *American Journal of Cardiology* 98, no. 8 (Oct. 15, 2006): 1069–72 (ePUB, Aug. 28, 2006).

11. L. H. Goldstein, L. Atkins, S. Landau, R. Brown, and P. N. Leigh, "Predictors of Psychological Distress in Carers of People with Amyotrophic Lateral Sclerosis: A Longitudinal Study," *Psychological Medicine* 36, no. 6 (June 2006): 865–75 (ePUB, Feb. 21, 2006).

12. B. Daneker, P. L. Kimmel, T. Ranich, and R. A. Peterson, "Depression and Marital Dissatisfaction in Patients with End-Stage Renal Disease and in Their Spouses," *American Journal of Kidney Disease* 38, no. 4 (Oct. 2001): 839–46.

13. J. L. Wolff, S. M. Dy, K. D. Frick, and J. D. Kasper, "End-of-Life Care: Findings from a National Survey of Informal Caregivers," *Archives of Internal Medicine* 167, no. 1 (Jan. 8, 2007): 40–46.

14. Y. Kim, D. K. Wellisch, R. L. Spillers, and C. Crammer, "Psychological Distress of Female Cancer Caregivers: Effects of Type of Cancer and Caregivers' Spirituality," *Support Care Cancer* 15, no. 12 (Dec. 2007): 1367–74.

15. L. A. Colgrove, Y. Kim, and N. Thompson, "The Effect of Spirituality and Gender on the Quality of Life of Spousal Caregivers of Cancer Survivors," *Annals of Behavioral Medicine* 33, no. 1 (Feb. 2007): 90–98.

16. Y. Kim, R. Schulz, and C. S. Carver, "Benefit-Finding in the Cancer Caregiving Experience," *Psychosomatic Medicine* 69, no. 3 (Apr. 2007): 283–91.

17. Oriah, "Invitation," *The Invitation* (San Francisco: HarperONE, 1999).

2. Care for Your Body

1. I. V. Zhdanova, R. J. Wurtman, M. M. Regan, J. A. Taylor, J. P. Shi, and O. U. Leclair. "Melatonin Treatment for Age-Related Insomnia." *Journal of Clinical Endocrinology and Metabolism* 86, no. 10 (Oct. 2001): 4727–30.
2. S. Bent, A. Padula, D. Moore, M. Patterson, and W. Mehling. "Valerian for Sleep: A Systematic Review and Meta-analysis." American Journal of Medicne 119, no. 12 (Dec. 2006):1005–12.

3. Stay Connected

1. The Wellness Community, www.thewellnesscommunity.org.

4. Follow a Daily Mindfulness Practice

1. Anonymous, "The Peace Prayer of Saint Francis," published by the Franciscan Archive, www.franciscan-archive.org/patriarcha/peace.html.

6. How Connection Heals

1. N. Hochhausen, E. M. Altmaier, R. McQuellon, S. M. Davies, E. Papadopolous, S. Carter, and J. Henslee Downey, "Social Support, Optimism, and Self-Efficacy Predict Physical and Emotional Well-being after Bone Marrow Transplantation," *Journal of Psychosocial Oncology* 25, no. 1 (2007): 87–101.
2. M. S. Thong, A. A. Kaptein, R. T. Krediet, E. W. Boeschoten, and F. W. Dekker, "Social Support Predicts Survival in Dialysis Patients," *Nephrology Dialysis and Transplantation* 22, no. 3 (Mar. 2007): 845–50 (ePUB, Dec. 12, 2006).
3. X. Zhang, S. L. Norris, E. W. Gregg, and G. Beckle, "Social Support and Mortality among Older Persons with Diabetes," *Diabetes Education* 33, no. 2 (Mar.–Apr. 2007): 273–81.
4. I. Ruiz Perez, J. Rodriguez Baño, M. A. Lopez Ruz, A. del Arco Jimenez, M. Causse Prados, J. Pasquau Liaño, P. Martin Rico, J. de la Torre Lima, J. L. Prada Pardal, M. Lopez Gomez, N. Muñoz, D. Morales, and M. Marcos, "Health-Related Quality of Life of Patients with HIV: Impact of Sociodemographic, Clinical and Psychosocial Factors," *Quality of Life Research* 14, no. 5 (June 2005): 1301–10.
5. E. L. Hurwitz, M. S. Goldstein, H. Morgenstern, and L. M. Chiang, "The Impact of Psychosocial Factors on Neck Pain and Disability Outcomes among Primary Care Patients: Results from the UCLA Neck Pain Study," *Disability Rehabilitation* 28, no. 21 (Nov. 15, 2006): 1319–29.
6. M. C. Davis, A. J. Zautra, and J. W. Reich, "Vulnerability to Stress among Women in Chronic Pain from Fibromyalgia and Osteoarthritis," *Annals of Behavioral Medicine* 23, no. 3 (Summer 2001): 215–26.

7. J. B. Prins, E. Bos, M. J. Huibers, P. Servaes, S. P. van der Werf, J. W. van der Meer, and G. Bleijenberg, "Social Support and the Persistence of Complaints in Chronic Fatigue Syndrome," *Psychotherapy Psychosomatics* 73, no. 3 (May–June 2004): 174–82.

8. W. Collinge, P. Yarnold, and E. Raskin, "Use of Mind/Body Self-Healing Practice Predicts Positive Health Transition in Chronic Fatigue Syndrome: A Controlled Study," *Subtle Energies and Energy Medicine* 9, no. 3 (1998): 171–90.

9. G. S. Alarcon, J. Calvo-Alen, G. McGwin Jr., A. G. Uribe, S. M. Toloza, J. M. Roseman, M. Fernandez, B. J. Fessler, L. M. Vila, C. Ahn, F. K. Tan, and J. D. Reveille—LUMINA Study Group, "Systemic Lupus Erythematosus in a Multiethnic Cohort—LUMINA XXXV: Predictive Factors of High Disease Activity over Time," *Annals of Rheumatic Disease* 65, no. 9 (Sept. 2006): 1168–74.

10. L. Fyrand, T. Moum, A. Finset, and A. Glennås, "The Effect of Social Network Intervention for Women with Rheumatoid Arthritis," *Family Process* 42, no. 1 (Spring 2003): 71–89.

11. E. Okkonen and H. Vanhanen, "Family Support, Living Alone, and Subjective Health of a Patient in Connection with a Coronary Artery Bypass Surgery," *Heart Lung* 35, no. 4 (July–Aug. 2006): 234–44.

12. B. J. Shen, C. P. McCreary, and H. F. Myers, "Independent and Mediated Contributions of Personality, Coping, Social Support, and Depressive Symptoms to Physical Functioning Outcome among Patients in Cardiac Rehabilitation," *Journal of Behavioral Medicine* 27, no. 1 (Feb. 2004): 39–62.

13. F. W. Craig, J. J. Lynch, and J. L. Quartner, "The Perception of Available Social Support Is Related to Reduced Cardiovascular Reactivity in Phase II Cardiac Rehabilitation Patients," *Integrative Physiological and Behavioral Science* 35, no. 4 (Oct.–Dec. 2000): 272–83.

14. A. B. Kornblith, J. E. Herndon, E. Zuckerman, C. M. Viscoli, R. I. Horwitz, M. R. Cooper, L. Harris, K. H. Tkaczuk, M. C. Perry, D. Budman, L. C. Norton, and J. Holland—Cancer and Leukemia Group B, "Social Support as a Buffer to the Psychological Impact of Stressful Life Events in Women with Breast Cancer," *Cancer* 91, no. 2 (Jan. 15, 2001): 443–54.

15. W. A. Bardwell, L. Natarajan, J. E. Dimsdale, C. L. Rock, J. E. Mortimer, K. Hollenbach, and J. P. Pierce, "Objective Cancer-Related Variables Are Not Associated with Depressive Symptoms in Women Treated for Early-Stage Breast Cancer," *Journal of Clinical Oncology* 24, no. 16 (June 1, 2006): 2420–27 (ePUB, May 1, 2006).

16. D. P. Kinsinger, F. J. Penedo, M. H. Antoni, J. R. Dahn, S. Lechner, and N. Schneiderman, "Psychosocial and Sociodemographic Correlates of Benefit-Finding in Men Treated for Localized Prostate Cancer," *Psychooncology* 15, no. 11 (Nov. 2006): 954–61.

17. K. J. Roberts, S. J. Lepore, and V. Helgeson, "Social-Cognitive Correlates of Adjustment to Prostate Cancer," *Psychooncology* 15, no. 3 (Mar. 2006): 183–92.

18. D. Shrock, R. F. Palmer, and B. Taylor, "Effects of a Psychosocial Intervention on Survival among Patients with Stage I Breast and Prostate Cancer: A Matched

Case-Control Study," *Alternative Therapies in Health and Medicine* 5, no. 3 (May 1999): 49–55.

19. I. C. Williams, "Emotional Health of Black and White Dementia Caregivers: A Contextual Examination," *The Journals of Gerontology, Series B, Pyschological Sciences and Social Sciences* 60, no. 6 (Nov. 2005): P287–P295.

20. D. L. Roth, M. S. Mittelman, O. J. Clay, A. Madan, and W. E. Haley, "Changes in Social Support as Mediators of the Impact of a Psychosocial Intervention for Spouse Caregivers of Persons with Alzheimer's Disease," *Psychology and Aging* 20, no. 4 (Dec. 2005): 634–44.

21. P. Drentea, O. J. Clay, D. L. Roth, and M. S. Mittelman, "Predictors of Improvement in Social Support: Five-Year Effects of a Structured Intervention for Caregivers of Spouses with Alzheimer's Disease," *Social Science and Medicine* 63, no. 4 (Aug. 2006): 957–67 (ePUB, Apr. 17, 2006).

22. E. McCullagh, G. Brigstocke, N. Donaldson, and L. Kalra, "Determinants of Caregiving Burden and Quality of Life in Caregivers of Stroke Patients," *Stroke* 36, no. 10 (Oct. 2005): 2181–86 (ePUB, Sept. 8, 2005).

23. M. S. Mittelman, W. E. Hale, O. J. Clay, and D. L. Roth, "Improving Caregiver Well-being Delays Nursing Home Placement of Patients with Alzheimer Disease," *Neurology* 67, no. 9 (Nov. 14, 2006): 1592–99.

24. B. Draper, G. Bowring, C. Thompson, J. Van Heyst, P. Conroy, and J. Thompson, "Stress in Caregivers of Aphasic Stroke Patients: A Randomized Controlled Trial," *Clinical Rehabilitation* 21, no. 2 (Feb. 2007): 122–30.

25. J. T. Newsom, K. S. Rook, M. Nishishiba, D. H. Sorkin, and T. L. Mahan, "Understanding the Relative Importance of Positive and Negative Social Exchanges: Examining Specific Domains and Appraisals," *The Journals of Gerontology, Series B, Psychological Sciences and Social Sciences* 60, no. 6 (Nov. 2005): P304–P312.

10. *Organize a Prayer Network*

1. For example, FreeConferenceCall.com.

11. *Attend (or Create) a Support Group with Other Couples*

1. The Wellness Community, www.thewellnesscommunity.org.

12. *The First Medicine*

1. C. A. Moyer, J. Rounds, and J. W. Hannum, "A Meta-Analysis of Massage Therapy Research," *Psychological Bulletin* 130, no. 1 (2004): 3–18.

2. B. R. Cassileth and A. J. Vickers, "Massage Therapy for Symptom Control: Outcome Study at a Major Cancer Center," *Journal of Pain and Symptom Management* 28, no. 3 (2004): 244–49.

3. S. S. Meek, "Effects of Slow Stroke Back Massage on Relaxation in Hospice Clients," *Image: Journal of Nursing Scholarship* 25 (1993): 17–21.

4. W. Collinge, J. Kahn, P. Yarnold, J. Astin, R. McCorkle, and S. Bauer-Wu. "Couples and Cancer: Outcomes of Brief Instruction in Massage and Touch Therapy to Build Caregiver Efficacy." *Journal of the Society for Integrative Oncology* 5, no. 4 (2007): 147–54.

5. *Touch, Caring and Cancer: Simple Instruction for Family and Friends* (DVD with manual). Collinge and Associates (2008). Available at www.PartnersinHealing.net.

6. D. Curties, "Could Massage Therapy Promote Cancer Metastasis?" *Massage Therapy* 39, no. 3 (2000): 83–90.

7. G. MacDonald, *Medicine Hands: Massage Therapy for People with Cancer* (Tallahassee, Fla.: Findhorn Press, 1999).

8. R. Gecsedi, "Massage Therapy for Patients with Cancer," *Clinical Journal of Oncology Nursing* 6, no. 1 (2002): 52–54.

9. W. Collinge, R. Wentworth, and S. Sabo, "Integrating Complementary Therapies into Community Mental Health Practice: An Exploration," *Journal of Alternative and Complementary Medicine* 11, no. 3 (June 2005): 569–74.

10. All information about acupressure points comes from Michael R. Gach, *Acupressure's Potent Points: A Guide to Self-Care for Common Ailments* (New York: Bantam Books, 1990).

13. Foot Massage

1 L. Grealish, A. Lomasney, and B. Whiteman, "Foot Massage. A Nursing Intervention to Modify the Distressing Symptoms of Pain and Nausea in Patients Hospitalized with Cancer," *Cancer Nursing* 23, no. 3 (2000): 237–43; N. L. Stephenson, S. P. Weinrich, and A. S. Tavakoli, "The Effects of Foot Reflexology on Anxiety and Pain in Patients with Breast and Lung Cancer," *Oncology Nursing Forum* 27, no. 1 (2000): 67–72; H. Hodgson, "Does Reflexology Impact on Cancer Patients' Quality of Life?" *Nursing Standard* 14, no. 31 (2000): 33–38.

19. Energy, Intention, and Healing

1. R. Kroiss, I. S. Fentiman, F. A. Helmond, J. Rymer, J. M. Foidart, N. Bundred, M. Mol-Arts, and E. Kubista, "The Effect of Tibolone in Postmenopausal Women Receiving Tamoxifen after Surgery for Breast Cancer: A Randomised, Double-Blind, Placebo-Controlled Trial," *BJOG: An International Journal of Obstetrics and Gynecology* 112, no. 2 (Feb. 2005): 228–33.

2. P. Wang, X. Hu, and B. Wu, "Displaying of the Infrared Radiant Track along Meridians on the Back of Human Body," *Chen Tzu Yen Chiu Acupuncture Research* 18, no. 2 (1993): 90–93, 89; and X. Hu, B. Wu, and P. Wang, "Displaying of Meridian Courses Traveling over Human Body Surface under Natural Conditions," *Chen Tzu Yen Chiu Acupuncture Research* 18, no. 2 (1993): 83–89.

3. Z. Yan, Y. Chi, P. Wang, J. Cheng, Y. Wang, Q. Shu, and G. Huang, "Studies on the Luminescence of Channels in Rats and Its Law of Changes with 'Syndromes' and Treatment of Acupuncture and Moxibustion," *Journal of Traditional Chinese Medicine* 12, no. 4 (Dec. 1992): 283–87.

4. A. Jackson, "Energetic Medicine: A New Science of Healing: Interview with Dr. Hiroshi Motoyama," *Share International Magazine* 11, no. 7 (1992): 5–7.

5. X. Hu, B. Wu, J. Xu, and J. Hao, "Studies on the Low Skin Impedance Points and the Features of Its Distribution along the Channels by Microcomputer: I. Observation on the Reliability of the Measurement," *Chen Tzu Yen Chiu Acupuncture Research* 15, no. 3 (1990): 232–38; and X. Hu, B. Wu, X. Huang, and J. Xu, "Computerized Plotting of Low Skin Impedance Points," *Journal of Traditional Chinese Medicine* 12, no. 4 (Dec. 1992): 277–82.

6. "Electronic Evidence of Auras, Chakras in UCLA Study," *Brain/Mind Bulletin* 3, no. 9 (Mar. 20, 1978); and R. Miller, "Bridging the Gap: An Interview with Valerie Hunt, Ed.D.," *Science of Mind* (Oct. 1983).

7. H. Motoyama and R. Brown, *Science and the Evolution of Consciousness: Chakras, Ki, and Psi* (Brookline, Mass.: Autumn Press, 1978), 93–98.

8. Jackson, "Energetic Medicine."

9. A. Cooperstein, "The Myths of Healing: A Summary of Research into Transpersonal Healing Experience," *Journal of Religion and Psychical Research* 15 (1992): 63–90.

10. M. Schlitz, "Intentionality in Healing: Mapping the Integration of Body, Mind, and Spirit," *Alternative Therapies in Health and Medicine* 1 (1995): 5, 119–20.

11. If you feel inspired to pursue training or instruction in specific methods of energy healing, there are many excellent training programs that are accessible to laypeople, and I would encourage you to explore them. See Additional Resources for information about opportunities for instruction.

12. N. Mackay, S. Hansen, and O. McFarlane, "Autonomic Nervous System Changes during Reiki Treatment: A Preliminary Study," *Journal of Alternative Complementary Medicine* 10, no. 6 (Dec. 2004): 1077–81.

13. K. D. Lafreniere, B. Mutus, S. Cameron, M. Tannous, M. Giannotti, H. Abu-Zahra, and E. Laukkanen, "Effects of Therapeutic Touch on Biochemical and Mood Indicators in Women," *Journal of Alternative Complementary Medicine* 5, no. 4 (Aug. 1999): 367–70.

14. E. Keller and V. M. Bzdek, "Effects of Therapeutic Touch on Tension Headache Pain," *Nursing Research* 35, no. 2 (Mar.–Apr. 1986): 101–6.

15. S. D. Peck, "The Efficacy of Therapeutic Touch for Improving Functional Ability in Elders with Degenerative Arthritis," *Nursing Science Quarterly* 11, no. 3 (Fall 1998): 123–32.

16. A. Gordon, J. H. Merenstein, F. D'Amico, and D. Hudgens, "The Effects of Therapeutic Touch on Patients with Osteoarthritis of the Knee," *Journal of Family Practice* 47, no. 4 (Oct. 1998): 271–77.

17. B. Denison, "Touch the Pain Away: New Research on Therapeutic Touch and Persons with Fibromyalgia Syndrome," *Holistic Nursing Practice* 18, no. 3 (May–June 2004): 142–51.

18. T. C. Meehan, "Therapeutic Touch and Postoperative Pain: A Rogerian Research Study," *Nursing Science Quarterly* 6, no. 2 (Summer 1993): 69–78.

19. C. Cox and J. Hayes, "Physiologic and Psychodynamic Responses to the Administration of Therapeutic Touch in Critical Care," *Complementary Therapies in Nursing and Midwifery* 5, no. 3 (June 1999): 87–92.

20. J. G. Turner, A. J. Clark, D. K. Gauthier, and M. Williams, "The Effect of Therapeutic Touch on Pain and Anxiety in Burn Patients," *Journal of Advances in Nursing* 28, no. 1 (July 1998): 10–20.

21. A. G. Shore, "Long-Term Effects of Energetic Healing on Symptoms of Psychological Depression and Self-Perceived Stress," *Alternative Therapies in Health and Medicine* 10, no. 3 (May–June 2004): 42–48.

22. J. F. Quinn, "Therapeutic Touch as Energy Exchange: Testing the Theory," *Advances in Nursing Science* 6, no. 2 (Jan. 1984): 42–49.

23. J. A. Simington and G. P. Laing, "Effects of Therapeutic Touch on Anxiety in the Institutionalized Elderly," *Clinical Nursing Research* 2, no. 4 (Nov. 1993): 438–50.

24. C. N. Larden, M. L. Palmer, and P. Janssen, "Efficacy of Therapeutic Touch in Treating Pregnant Inpatients Who Have a Chemical Dependency," *Journal of Holistic Nursing* 22, no. 4 (Dec. 2004): 320–32.

25. M. Giasson and L. Bouchard, "Effect of Therapeutic Touch on the Well-being of Persons with Terminal Cancer," *Journal of Holistic Nursing* 16, no. 3 (Sept. 1998): 383–98.

26. J. A. Roscoe, S. E. Matteson, K. M. Mustian, D. Padmanaban, and G. R. Morrow, "Treatment of Radiotherapy-Induced Fatigue through a Nonpharmacological Approach," *Integrative Cancer Therapies* 4, no. 1 (Mar. 2005): 8–13.

   C. A. Cook, J. F. Guerrerio, and V. E. Slater, "HT and Quality of Life in Women Receiving Radiation Treatment for Cancer: A Randomized Controlled Trial," *Alternative Therapies in Health and Medicine* 10, no. 3 (May–June 2004): 34–41.

27. K. Olson, J. Hanson, and M. Michaud, "A Phase II Trial of Reiki for the Management of Pain in Advanced Cancer Patients," *Journal of Pain and Symptom Management* 26, no. 5 (Nov. 2003): 990–97.

28. J. Post-White, M. E. Kinney, K. Savik, J. B. Gau, C. Wilcox, and I. Lerner, "Therapeutic Massage and HT Improve Symptoms in Cancer," *Integrative Cancer Therapies* 2, no. 4 (Dec. 2003): 332–44.

29. D. L. Woods, R. F. Craven, and J. Whitney, "The Effect of Therapeutic Touch on Behavioral Symptoms of Persons with Dementia," *Alternative Therapies in Health and Medicine* 11, no. 1 (Jan.–Feb. 2005): 66–74.

30. M. Giasson, G. Leroux, H. Tardif, and L. Bouchard, "Therapeutic Touch," *L'Infirmiere du Quebec* 6, no. 6 (July–Aug. 1999): 38–47.

20. Balancing Energy

1. J. A. Roscoe, S. E. Matteson, K. M. Mustian, D. Padmanaban, and G. R. Morrow, "Treatment of Radiotherapy-Induced Fatigue through a Nonpharmacological Approach," *Integrative Cancer Therapies* 4, no. 1 (Mar. 2005): 8–13.
2. American Polarity Therapy Association, www.polaritytherapy.org.

23. Chakra Connection

1. W. B. Joy, *Joy's Way* (Los Angeles: J. P. Tarcher, 1979).

27. Never Beyond Reach

1. L. Dossey, *Reinventing Medicine: Beyond Mind-Body to a New Era of Healing* (New York: HarperCollins, 1999).
2. "Spooky Teleportation Study Brings Future Closer," Reuters, Oct. 22, 1998.
3. J. Grinberg-Zylberbaum, M. Delaflor, M. E. Sanchez, et al., "Human Communication and the Electrophysiological Activity of the Brain," *Subtle Energies* 3, no. 3 (1992): 25–43.
4. H. Walach, "Theory and Apory in Healing Research: 'Influence' versus 'Correlational' Models," *Subtle Energies & Energy Medicine* 11, no. 2 (2000): 189–206.
5. Ibid., 201.
6. Ibid.
7. Ibid., 202.
8. J. Solfvin, E. Leskowitz, and D. J. Benor, "Questions Concerning the Work of Daniel P. Wirth," *Journal of Complementary and Alternative Medicine* 11, no. 6 (Dec. 2005): 949–50.
9. F. Sicher, E. Targ, D. Moore II, and H. S. Smith, "A Randomized, Double-Blind Study of the Effects of Distant Healing in a Population with Advanced AIDS: Report of a Small Scale Study," *Western Journal of Medicine* 169, no. 6 (Dec. 1998): 356–63 (republished in *Subtle Energies & Energy Medicine* 9, no. 20 [2000]: 83–100).

    M. W. Krucoff, S. W. Crater, D. Gallup, J. C. Blankenship, M. Cuffe, M. Guarneri, R. A. Krieger, V. R. Kshettry, K. Morris, M. Oz, A. Pichard, M. H. Sketch Jr., H. G. Koenig, D. Mark, and K. L. Lee, "Music, Imagery, Touch, and Prayer as Adjuncts to Interventional Cardiac Care: The Monitoring and Actualisation of Noetic Trainings (MANTRA) II Randomised Study," *Lancet* 366, no. 9481 (July 16–22, 2005): 211–17.
10. R. Byrd, "Positive Therapeutic Effects of Intercessory Prayer in a Coronary Care Unit Population," *Southern Medical Journal* 81 (1988): 826–29.
11. M. Schlitz and W. Braud, "Distant Intentionality and Healing: Assessing the Evidence," *Alternative Therapies in Health and Medicine* 3, no. 6 (Nov. 1997): 62–73.

12. J. Achterberg, K. Cooke, T. Richards, L. J. Standish, L. Kozak, and J. Lake, "Evidence for Correlations between Distant Intentionality and Brain Function in Recipients: A Functional Magnetic Resonance Imaging Analysis," *Journal of Complementary and Alternative Medicine* 11, no. 6 (Dec. 2005): 965–71.

13. C. C. Crawford, A. G. Sparber, and W. B. Jonas, "A Systematic Review of the Quality of Research on Hands-On and Distance Healing: Clinical and Laboratory Studies," *Alternative Therapies in Health and Medicine* 9, suppl. 3 (May–June 2003): A96–A104.

    J. A. Astin, E. Harkness, and E. Ernst, "The Efficacy of 'Distant Healing': A Systematic Review of Randomized Trials," *Annals of Internal Medicine* 132, no. 11 (June 6, 2000): 903–10.

    L. Roberts, I. Ahmed, and S. Hall, "Intercessory Prayer for the Alleviation of Ill Health," *Cochrane Database Systematic Reviews,* no. 2 (2000): CD000368.

14. S. R. Walker, J. S. Tonigan, W. R. Miller, S. Corner, and L. Kahlich, "Intercessory Prayer in the Treatment of Alcohol Abuse and Dependence: A Pilot Investigation," *Alternative Therapies in Health and Medicine* 3, no. 6 (Nov. 1997): 79–86.

15. J. Mathai and A. Bourne, "Pilot Study Investigating the Effect of Intercessory Prayer in the Treatment of Child Psychiatric Disorders," *Australasian Psychiatry* 12, no. 4 (Dec. 2004): 386–89.

16. N. C. Abbot, E. F. Harkness, C. Stevinson, F. P. Marshall, D. A. Conn, and E. Ernst, "Spiritual Healing as a Therapy for Chronic Pain: A Randomized, Clinical Trial," *Pain* 91, nos. 1–2 (Mar. 2001): 79–89.

17. E. F. Harkness, N. C. Abbot, and E. Ernst, "A Randomized Trial of Distant Healing for Skin Warts," *American Journal of Medicine* 108, no. 6 (Apr. 15, 2000): 448–52.

18. M. Ebneter, M. Binder, O. Kristof, H. Walach, and R. Saller, "Distant Healing and Diabetes Mellitus: A Pilot Study," *Forsch Komplementarmed Klass Naturheilkd* 9, no. 1 (Feb. 2002): 22–30.

19. B. Greyson, "Distance Healing of Patients with Major Depression," *Journal of Scientific Exploration* 10, no. 4 (1996): 447–65.

20. J. Tloczynski and S. Fritzsch, "Intercessory Prayer in Psychological Well-being: Using a Multiple-Baseline, across-Subjects Design," *Psychological Reports* 91, no. 3, pt. 1 (Dec. 2002): 731–41.

21. P. J. Collipp, "The Efficacy of Prayer: A Triple-Blind Study," *Medical Times* 97, no. 5 (May 1969): 201–4.

22. Byrd, "Positive Therapeutic Effects of Intercessory Prayer in a Coronary Care Unit Population."

    W. S. Harris, M. Gowda, J. W. Kolb, C. P. Strychacz, J. L. Vacek, P. G. Jones, A. Forker, J. H. O'Keefe, and B. D. McCallister, "A Randomized, Controlled Trial of the Effects of Remote, Intercessory Prayer on Outcomes in Patients Admitted to the Coronary Care Unit," *Archives of Internal Medicine* 159, no. 19 (Oct. 25, 1999): 2273–78 (erratum in *Archives of Internal Medicine* 160, no. 12 [June 26, 2000]: 1878).

23. H. Benson, J. A. Dusek, J. B. Sherwood, P. Lam, C. F. Bethea, W. Carpenter, S. Levitsky, P. C. Hill, D. W. Clem Jr., M. K. Jain, D. Drumel, S. L. Kopecky, P. S. Mueller, D. Marek, S. Rollins, and P. L. Hibberd, "Study of the Therapeutic Effects of Intercessory Prayer (STEP) in Cardiac Bypass Patients: A Multicenter Randomized Trial of Uncertainty and Certainty of Receiving Intercessory Prayer," *American Heart Journal* 151, no. 4 (Apr. 2006): 934–42.

24. Krucoff et al., "Music, Imagery, Touch, and Prayer as Adjuncts to Interventional Cardiac Care."

    J. M. Aviles, S. E. Whelan, D. A. Hernke, B. A. Williams, K. E. Kenny, W. M. O'Fallon, and S. L. Kopecky, "Intercessory Prayer and Cardiovascular Disease Progression in a Coronary Care Unit Population: A Randomized Controlled Trial," *Mayo Clinic Proceedings* 76, no. 12 (Dec. 2001): 1192–98.

25. R. M. Miller, "Study on the Effectiveness of Remote Mental Healing," *Medical Hypotheses* 8, no. 5 (May 1982): 481–90.

26. Sicher, Targ, Moore 2nd, and Smith, "Randomized Double-Blind Study of the Effect of Distant Healing in a Population with Advanced AIDS."

27. J. A. Astin, J. Stone, D. I. Abrams, D. H. Moore, P. Couey, R. Buscemi, and E. Targ, "The Efficacy of Distant Healing for Human Immunodeficiency Virus—Results of a Randomized Trial," *Alternative Therapies in Health and Medicine* 12, no. 6 (Nov.–Dec. 2006): 36–41.

28. R. L. Harmon and M. A. Myers, "Prayer and Meditation as Medical Therapies," *Physical and Medical Rehabilitation Clinics of North America* 10, no. 3 (Aug. 1999): 651–62; J. S. Levin, "How Prayer Heals: A Theoretical Model," *Alternative Therapies in Health and Medicine* 2, no. 1 (Jan. 1996): 66–73; and A. L. Ai, R. E. Dunkle, C. Peterson, and S. F. Bolling, "The Role of Private Prayer in Psychological Recovery among Mid-life and Aged Patients Following Cardiac Surgery," *Gerontologist* 38, no. 5 (Oct. 1998): 591–601; H. Benson, J. Beary, and M. Carol, "The Relaxation Response," *Psychiatry* 37 (1974): 37–46; H. Benson, *Beyond the Relaxation Response* (New York: Berkley Books, 1985); S. W. Lazar, G. Bush, R. L. Gollub, G. L. Fricchione, G. Khalsa, and H. Benson, "Functional Brain Mapping of the Relaxation Response and Meditation," *Neuroreport* 11, no. 7 (May 15, 2000): 1581–85; G. Stefano, G. Fricchione, B. Slingsby, and H. Benson, "The Placebo Effect and Relaxation Response: Neural Processes and Their Coupling to Constitutive Nitric Oxide," *Brain Research Reviews* 35 (2001): 1–19; L. S. Eller, "Guided Imagery Interventions for Symptom Management," *Annual Reviews of Nursing Research* 17 (1999): 57–84; E. Ernst and N. Kanji, "Autogenic Training for Stress and Anxiety: A Systematic Review," *Complementary Therapies in Medicine* 8, no. 2 (June 2000): 106–10; S. L. Shapiro, G. E. Schwartz, and G. Bonner, "Effects of Mindfulness-Based Stress Reduction on Medical and Premedical Students," *Journal of Behavioral Medicine* 21, no. 6 (Dec. 1998): 581–99; J. Kabat-Zinn, A. O. Massion, J. Kristeller, L. G. Peterson, K. E. Fletcher, L. Obert, W. R. Lenderking, and S. F. Santorelli, "Effectiveness of a Meditation-Based Stress Reduction Program in the Treat-

ment of Anxiety Disorders," *American Journal of Psychiatry* 149, no. 7 (July 1992): 936–43; J. Kabat-Zinn, E. Wheeler, T. Light, A. Skillings, M. J. Scharf, T. G. Cropley, D. Hosmer, and J. D. Bernhard, "Influence of a Mindfulness Meditation-Based Stress Reduction Intervention on Rates of Skin Clearing in Patients with Moderate to Severe Psoriasis Undergoing Phototherapy (UVB) and Photochemotherapy (PUVA)," *Psychosomatic Medicine* 60, no. 5 (Sep.–Oct. 1998): 625–32; A. O. Massion, J. Teas, J. R. Hebert, M. D. Wertheimer, and J. Kabat-Zinn, "Meditation, Melatonin and Breast/Prostate Cancer: Hypothesis and Preliminary Data," *Medical Hypotheses* 44, no. 1 (Jan. 1995): 39–46; J. J. Miller, K. Fletcher, and J. Kabat-Zinn, "Three-Year Follow-up and Clinical Implications of a Mindfulness Meditation-Based Stress Reduction Intervention in the Treatment of Anxiety Disorders," *General Hospital Psychiatry* 17, no. 3 (May 1995): 192–200; C. Cunningham, S. Brown, and J. C. Kaski, "Effects of Transcendental Meditation on Symptoms and Electrocardiographic Changes in Patients with Cardiac Syndrome X," *American Journal of Cardiology* 85, no. 5 (Mar. 1, 2000): 653–55, A10; G. A. Tooley, S. M. Armstrong, T. R. Norman, and A. Sali, "Acute Increases in Night-time Plasma Melatonin Levels Following a Period of Meditation," *Biological Psychology* 53, no. 1 (May 2000): 69–78; F. Travis, J. J. Tecce, and J. Guttman, "Cortical Plasticity, Contingent Negative Variation, and Transcendent Experiences during Practice of the Transcendental Meditation Technique," *Biological Psychology* 55, no. 1 (Nov. 2000): 41–55.

29. S. ÓLaoire, "An Experimental Study of the Effects of Distant, Intercessory Prayer on Self-Esteem, Anxiety, and Depression," *Alternative Therapies in Health and Medicine* 3, no. 6 (1997): 19–53.

30. M. Schlitz and E. Targ, personal communication.

31. A. Cooperstein, "The Myths of Healing: A Summary of Research into Transpersonal Healing Experience," *Journal of Religion and Psychical Research* 15 (1992): 63–90.

32. C. Longaker, *Facing Death and Finding Hope: A Guide to the Emotional and Spiritual Care of the Dying* (New York: Doubleday, 1997).

33. L. G. Underwood, "The Human Experience of Compassionate Love: Conceptual Mapping and Data from Selected Studies," in S. G. Post, L. G. Underwood, J. P. Schloss, and W. B. Hurlbut, eds., *Altruism and Altruistic Love: Science, Philosophy, and Religion in Dialogue* (Oxford, U.K.: Oxford University Press, 2002), 72–88.

34. S. Krippner, unpublished manuscript. Dr. Krippner is a pioneer in the study of consciousness and a professor at the Saybrook Graduate School in San Francisco.

28. Transforming Suffering

1. S. Rinpoche, *The Tibetan Book of Living and Dying* (San Francisco: HarperSanFrancisco, 1992), 204–5.

34. Well-Chosen Words

1. S. Manne, M. Sherman, S. Ross, J. Ostroff, R. E. Heyman, and K. Fox, "Couples' Support-Related Communication, Psychological Distress, and Relationship Satisfaction among Women with Early Stage Breast Cancer," *Journal of Consulting and Clinical Psychology* 72, no. 4 (Aug. 2004): 660–70.

2. S. Manne, J. Ostroff, C. Rini, K. Fox, L. Goldstein, and G. Grana, "The Interpersonal Process Model of Intimacy: The Role of Self-Disclosure, Partner Disclosure, and Partner Responsiveness in Interactions between Breast Cancer Patients and Their Partners," *Journal of Family Psychology* 18, no. 4 (Dec. 2004): 589–99.

3. N. Pistrang and C. Barker, "The Partner Relationship in Psychological Response to Breast Cancer," *Social Science and Medicine* 40, no. 6 (Mar. 1995): 789–97.

4. H. Badr and L. K. Acitelli, "Dyadic Adjustment in Chronic Illness: Does Relationship Talk Matter?" *Journal of Family Psychology* 19, no. 3 (Sept. 2005): 465–69.

5. J. Normand, J. C. Lasry, R. G. Margolese, J. C. Perry, and D. Fleiszer, "Marital Communication and Depressive Symptoms in Couples in Which the Woman Has Cancer of the Breast," *Bulletin of Cancer* 91, no. 2 (Feb. 2004): 193–99.

6. B. L. Walker, "Adjustment of Husbands and Wives to Breast Cancer," *Cancer Practice* 5, no. 2 (Mar.–Apr. 1997): 92–98.

7. L. S. Porter, F. J. Keefe, H. Hurwitz, and M. Faber, "Disclosure between Patients with Gastrointestinal Cancer and Their Spouses," *Psychooncology* 14, no. 12 (Dec. 2005): 1030–42.

8. T. R. Newton-John and A. C. Williams, "Chronic Pain Couples: Perceived Marital Interactions and Pain Behaviours," *Pain* 123, nos. 1–2 (July 2006): 53–63 (ePUB, Mar. 24, 2006).

9. M. Dorval, S. Guay, M. Mondor, B. Mâsse, M. Falardeau, A. Robidoux, L. Deschênes, and E. Maunsell, "Couples Who Get Closer after Breast Cancer: Frequency and Predictors in a Prospective Investigation," *Journal of Clinical Oncology* 23, no. 15 (May 20, 2005): 3588–96.

10. S. Manne, J. Ostroff, G. Winkel, L. Goldstein, K. Fox, and G. Grana, "Posttraumatic Growth after Breast Cancer: Patient, Partner, and Couple Perspectives," *Psychosomatic Medicine* 66, no. 3 (May–June 2004): 442–54.

11. M. L. Brecht, K. Dracup, D. K. Moser, and B. Riegel, "The Relationship of Marital Quality and Psychosocial Adjustment to Heart Disease," *Journal of Cardiovascular Nursing* 9, no. 1 (Oct. 1994): 74–85.

12. M. Svedlund and E. Danielson, "Myocardial Infarction: Narrations by Afflicted Women and Their Partners of Lived Experiences in Daily Life Following an Acute Myocardial Infarction," *Journal of Clinical Nursing* 13, no. 4 (May 2004): 438–46; and M. Svedlund and I. Axelsson, "Acute Myocardial Infarction in Middle-Aged Women: Narrations from the Patients and Their Partners during Rehabilitation," *Intensive Critical Care Nursing* 16, no. 4 (Aug. 2000): 256–65.

13. J. Gosling and M. Oddy, "Rearranged Marriages: Marital Relationships after Head Injury," *Brain Injury* 13, no. 10 (Oct. 1999): 785–96.

14. S. L. Manne, J. Ostroff, G. Winkel, G. Grana, and K. Fox, "Partner Unsupportive Responses, Avoidant Coping, and Distress among Women with Early Stage Breast Cancer: Patient and Partner Perspectives," *Health Psychology* 24, no. 6 (Nov. 2005): 635–41.

15. S. L. Manne, J. S. Ostroff, T. R. Norton, K. Fox, L. Goldstein, and G. Grana, "Cancer-Related Relationship Communication in Couples Coping with Early Stage Breast Cancer," *Psychooncology* 15, no. 3 (Mar. 2006): 234–47.

16. M. Losada and E. Heaphy, "Positivity and Connectivity," *American Behavioral Scientist* 47, no. 6 (2004): 740–65.

17. J. M. Gottman, *Why Marriages Succeed or Fail* (New York: Simon & Schuster, 1994).

35. *Sharing Heart's Intentions*

1. H. Wiesendanger, L. Werthmuller, K. Reuter, and H. Walach, "Chronically Ill Patients Treated by Spiritual Healing Improve in Quality of Life: Results of a Randomized Waiting-List Controlled Study," *Journal of Alternative and Complementary Therapies* 7, no. 1 (Feb. 2001): 45–51.

38. *Sleeping Separately*

1. H. Moldofsky, "Management of Sleep Disorders in Fibromyalgia," *Rheumatic Disease Clinics of North America* 28, no. 2 (May 2002): 353–65.

2. M. T. Smith, R. R. Edwards, U. D. McCann, and J. A. Haythornthwaite, "The Effects of Sleep Deprivation on Pain Inhibition and Spontaneous Pain in Women," *Sleep* 30, no. 4 (Apr. 1, 2007): 494–505.

3. H. Moldofsky, "Sleep and Pain," *Sleep Medicine* 5, no. 5 (Oct. 2001): 385–96.

4. A. Dzaja, S. Arber, J. Hislop, M. Kerkhofs, C. Kopp, T. Pollmächer, P. Polo-Kantola, D. J. Skene, P. Stenuit, I. Tobler, and T. Porkka-Heiskanen, "Women's Sleep in Health and Disease," *Journal of Psychiatric Research* 39, no. 1 (Jan. 2005): 55–76.

39. *The Art of the Bath*

1. J. Pizzorno and M. Murray, *Texbook of Natural Medicine* (New York: Churchill Livingstone, 1999).

2. K. Ammer and P. Melnizky, "Medicinal Baths for Treatment of Generalized Fibromyalgia," *Forsch Komplementarmed* 6, no. 2 (Apr. 1999): 80–85.

3. The Burton Goldberg Group, *Alternative Medicine: The Definitive Guide* (Puyallup, Wash.: Future Medicine, 1993).

40. Foot Bathing

1. *Caution:* Hot footbaths should be avoided by people with arteriosclerosis, Buerger's disease, or diabetes mellitus.

41. Food for the Soul

1. D. A. Zellner, S. Loaiza, Z. Gonzalez, J. Pita, J. Morales, D. Pecora, and A. Wolf, "Food Selection Changes under Stress," *Physiology and Behavior* 87, no. 4 (Apr. 15, 2006): 789–93 (ePUB, Mar. 6, 2006).
2. M. F. Dallman, N. Pecoraro, S. F. Akana, S. E. La Fleur, F. Gomez, H. Houshyar, M. E. Bell, S. Bhatnagar, K. D. Laugero, and S. Manalo, "Chronic Stress and Obesity: A New View of 'Comfort Food,'" *Proceedings of the National Academy of Sciences USA* 100, no. 20 (Sept. 30, 2003): 11696–701 (ePUB, Sept. 15, 2003).

   N. Pecoraro, F. Reyes, F. Gomez, A. Bhargava, and M. F. Dallman, "Chronic Stress Promotes Palatable Feeding, Which Reduces Signs of Stress: Feedforward and Feedback Effects of Chronic Stress," *Endocrinology* 145, no. 8 (Aug. 2004): 3754–62 (ePUB, May 13, 2004).
3. L. Dubé, J. L. LeBel, and J. Lu, "Affect Asymmetry and Comfort Food Consumption," *Physiology and Behavior* 86, no. 4 (Nov. 15, 2005): 559–67 (ePUB, Oct. 4, 2005).
4. B. Wansink, M. M. Cheney, and N. Chan, "Exploring Comfort Food Preferences across Age and Gender," *Physiology and Behavior* 79, nos. 4–5 (Sept. 2003): 739–47.
5. T. L. Dillinger, P. Barriga, S. Escárcega, M. Jimenez, D. Salazar Lowe, and L. E. Grivetti, "Food of the Gods: Cure for Humanity? A Cultural History of the Medicinal and Ritual Use of Chocolate," *Journal of Nutrition* 130, suppl. 8S (Aug. 2000): S2057–S2072.
6. D. Taubert, R. Roesen, C. Lehmann, N. Jung, and E. Schömig, "Effects of Low Habitual Cocoa Intake on Blood Pressure and Bioactive Nitric Oxide: A Randomized Controlled Trial," *Journal of the American Medical Association* 298, no. 1 (July 4, 2007): 49–60.
7. D. Grassi, S. Necozione, C. Lippi, G. Croce, L. Valeri, P. Pasqualetti, G. Desideri, J. B. Blumberg, and C. Ferri, "Cocoa Reduces Blood Pressure and Insulin Resistance and Improves Endothelium-Dependent Vasodilation in Hypertensives," *Hypertension* 46, no. 2 (Aug. 2005): 398–405 (ePUB, July 18, 2005).
8. Y. Wan, J. A. Vinson, T. D. Etherton, J. Proch, S. A. Lazarus, and P. M. Kris-Etherton, "Effects of Cocoa Powder and Dark Chocolate on LDL Oxidative Susceptibility and Prostaglandin Concentrations in Humans," *American Journal of Clinical Nutrition* 74, no. 5 (Nov. 2001): 596–602.
9. M. B. Engler, M. M. Engler, C. Y. Chen, M. J. Malloy, A. Browne, E. Y. Chiu, H. K. Kwak, P. Milbury, S. M. Paul, J. Blumberg, and M. L. Mietus-Snyder,

"Flavonoid-Rich Dark Chocolate Improves Endothelial Function and Increases Plasma Epicatechin Concentrations in Healthy Adults," *Journal of the American College of Nutrition* 23, no. 3 (June 2004): 197–204.

10. D. Grassi, C. Lippi, S. Necozione, G. Desideri, and C. Ferri, "Short-Term Administration of Dark Chocolate Is Followed by a Significant Increase in Insulin Sensitivity and a Decrease in Blood Pressure in Healthy Persons," *American Journal of Clinical Nutrition* 81, no. 3 (Mar. 2005): 611–14.

11. C. Jourdain, G. Tenca, A. Deguercy, P. Troplin, and D. Poelman, "In-vitro Effects of Polyphenols from Cocoa and Beta-Sitosterol on the Growth of Human Prostate Cancer and Normal Cells," *European Journal of Cancer Prevention* 15, no. 4 (Aug. 2006): 353–61.

D. Ramljak, L. J. Romanczyk, L. J. Metheny-Barlow, N. Thompson, V. Knezevic, M. Galperin, A. Ramesh, and R. B. Dickson, "Pentameric Procyanidin from Theobroma Cacao Selectively Inhibits Growth of Human Breast Cancer Cells," *Molecular Cancer Therapies* 4, no. 4 (Apr. 2005): 537–46.

12. "Dark Chocolate Eases M.E. [myalgic encephalomyelitis] Symptoms," METRO.co.uk, Dec. 18, 2006, www.metro.co.uk/news/article.html?in_article_id=29789&in_page_id=34.

42. The Art of Tea

1. J. Pizzorno and M. Murray, *Texbook of Natural Medicine,* vol. 1. (New York: Churchill Livingstone, 1999), 625.

N. Khan and H. Mukhtar, "Tea Polyphenols for Health Promotion," *Life Sciences* 81, no. 7 (July 26, 2007): 519–33.

2. R. Cooper, D. J. Morre, and D. M. Morre, "Medicinal Benefits of Green Tea," pt. 1, "Review of Noncancer Health Benefits," *Journal of Alternative Complementary Medicine* 11, no. 3 (June 2005): 521–28.

R. Cooper, D. J. Morre, and D. M. Morre, "Medicinal Benefits of Green Tea," pt. 2, "Review of Anticancer Properties," *Journal of Alternative Complementary Medicine* 11, no. 4 (Aug. 2005): 639–52.

3. M. Lorenz, N. Jochmann, A. von Krosigk, P. Martus, G. Baumann, K. Stangl, and V. Stangl, "Addition of Milk Prevents Vascular Protective Effects of Tea," *European Heart Journal* 28, no. 2 (Jan. 2007): 219–23 (ePUB, Jan. 9, 2007).

4. If you don't have a filter, consider buying an inexpensive carbon filter unit that can be attached to the faucet. This makes a real difference in the quality of the water that will go into the tea.

DVD Program

1. Winner of two 2008 Telly Awards in the categories of Health and Wellness and Social Issues.

Index

About the Author

WILLIAM COLLINGE, PHD, is a researcher and consultant in the
fields of behavioral medicine and caregiving. He has over twenty years
experience working with individuals, couples, and families living with
the challenges of cancer, HIV/AIDS, chronic fatigue syndrome, fibromyalgia, and other conditions. His previous books include *The American
Holistic Health Association Complete Guide to Alternative Medicine,
Recovering from Chronic Fatigue Syndrome,* and *Subtle Energy.*

As president of Collinge and Associates he directs studies on complementary therapies and caregiving sponsored by the National Institutes of
Health. These have included the Elder Healer Project, the Fibromyalgia
Wellness Project, and the Caring and Cancer Project that led to publica-
tion of the DVD program *Touch, Caring and Cancer: Simple Instruction for Family and Friends.* He is also a scientific review consultant for
government research programs in complementary therapies, cancer, and
other health conditions. William has led retreats and workshops internationally and is committed to helping people explore their healing abilities, both personally and in their relationships. For more information
visit www.collinge.org.